ID599648

YOUR HEART

Complete Information for the Family

Other Books by the Same Authors

AUSCULTATION OF THE HEART
  by Bernard L. Segal and William Likoff
CORONARY HEART DISEASE
  edited by William Likoff and John H. Moyer
ENGINEERING IN THE PRACTICE OF MEDICINE
  edited by Bernard L. Segal and David G. Kilpatrick
THE FAMILY BOOK OF PREVENTIVE MEDICINE
  by Benjamin F. Miller and Lawrence Galton
THE LABORATORY OF THE BODY
  by Lawrence Galton
THEORY AND PRACTICE OF AUSCULTATION
  edited by Bernard L. Segal, William Likoff, and John H. Moyer

WILLIAM LIKOFF, M.D.
BERNARD SEGAL, M.D.
and LAWRENCE GALTON

YOUR HEART

Complete Information for the Family

A PHILADELPHIA BULLETIN BOOK

J. B. Lippincott Company
Philadelphia and New York

Copyright © 1972 by William Likoff, M.D., Bernard Segal, M.D., and Lawrence Galton

Printed in the United States of America

U.S. Library of Congress Cataloging in Publication Data

Likoff, William.
        Your heart; complete information for the family.

        "A Philadelphia bulletin book."
        1. Heart. 2. Heart—Diseases. I. Segal, Bernard L., joint author. II. Galton, Lawrence, joint author. III. Title. [DNLM: 1. Cardiology—Popular works. WG 113 L727y 1972 (P)]
RC667.L56   616.1'2   75-37607
ISBN-0-397-00789-2

The diet plan presented in the appendix of this book is used with the gracious permission of the American Heart Association.

To Geoffrey, Jodi, David, Heidi and Jonathan
and to all children, who we hope will be spared a need
for this book.

WILLIAM LIKOFF, M.D.
BERNARD SEGAL, M.D.

To Kit, Jill, Jeremy, their mother and mine.

LAWRENCE GALTON

Contents

Introduction

At some point in life almost all of us receive a shock: we—or a relative or friend—have, or think we have, heart disease.

Even the suspicion of heart disease can provoke tremendous anxiety. For far too few of us realize that in recent years—mostly in the last decade or two—there have been remarkable advances in the treatment of most diseases affecting the heart. In some of these matters, progress has gone beyond prophecy.

There is a practical need to bridge the gap between what medicine has learned and what the patient and the patient's family understand about the possibilities of treatment. Often, understanding may mean the difference between despair and great hope, between invalidism and productive living, even between death and life.

Every physician would like to provide such understanding. But at the end of a long examination session—history-taking, a physical, electrocardiographic and other tests—the patient and family may be unprepared or too upset to grasp all the facts the physician tries to impart. The authors are very much aware of this problem. Two of us are practicing cardiologists and face the problem daily.

The human body has been called a wonderful machine, as of course it is—more wonderful than most of us realize. Virtually every part of it has remarkable features.

Human bone, for example, is as strong as cast iron, yet much lighter and more flexible. When a pole vaulter lands from his vault, his thigh bones bear up under as much as 20,000 pounds of pressure per square inch.

A single square inch of human skin contains 15 feet of very small blood vessels, 72 feet of nerves and hundreds of receptors for pain, pressure, heat and cold.

The human eye can perceive light as weak as one hundred-trillionth of a watt, and the trained ear, without help from the eyes, can locate precisely eighteen different instruments in an orchestra from a distance of 50 feet.

Human muscles, too, have their remarkable aspects. There are more than 600 in the body, made up of 6 trillion fibers, each fiber about the size of a hair and capable of supporting 1,000 times its own weight. A British physiologist recently calculated that an average man's muscles can produce 0.4 horsepower—enough, given the right wing equipment, to allow him to fly.

The most important muscle of all, of course, is a very special one, the heart.

Man has always been fascinated by the heart. Some of the ancients viewed it as the seat not only of life but of intelligence and reasoning power. Even Aristotle held to that belief and looked on the brain as simply the cooling mechanism for the heart. Today we know that none of this is true: the heart is just a pump—but a remarkable one.

If you are a normal adult of average weight, your heart pumps at a rate of about 70 to 75 times each minute, between 10 and 12 pints of blood per minute—blood that makes its way through 50 feet of arteries and veins and 62,000 miles of capillaries. Your heart beats 4,200 times an hour, over 36 million times a year, more than 2½ billion times if yours is the average lifetime.

The heart is not only a remarkable organ; it is a tough one.

We have really only begun to learn how tough it is. With this new knowledge, a new era is opening up even for those with severe heart problems.

Each year in the United States, 30,000 to 40,000 children—"blue babies" and others—are born with heart defects. Still other children develop trouble later, acquiring heart defects as a result of rheumatic-fever complications or other causes.

At one time the heart was considered the ultimate frontier of surgery, a frontier likely never to be crossed. But during the past two decades of important developments, surgeons, increasingly aware of the heart's intrinsic toughness, have been crossing the frontier more and more frequently, actually penetrating the heart to repair defects and, when necessary, replacing defective parts, such as valves, with artificial ones.

The heart may enlarge and eventually fail as a result of long-continued high blood pressure, but medical measures have been developed that are highly effective in combating this problem, so that many thousands of lives are being saved. In the last fifteen years the death rate from hypertensive heart disease has been cut almost in half. It can be cut further with measures now available. Even malignant hypertension—so called because it is a rapidly progressive form of high blood pressure which once killed 80 percent of its victims within a year—is being controlled with medication.

A major health problem is coronary heart disease, an affliction, resulting from the hardening and thickening, clogging and narrowing of the coronary arteries, which feed the heart muscle itself. But here, too, progress is being made—if not yet as much as we would like, at least much more than most people realize.

It was not until 1911 that the clinical pattern caused by closure of a coronary artery and subsequent destruction of a portion of heart muscle was first described, though the affliction has always been with us. Even in the 1920's and 1930's, coronary attacks were rarely diagnosed. If an individual died suddenly, unexpectedly, the verdict might be "a coronary." But if he became acutely ill and then recovered, it was often supposed that he could not have had a heart attack, or he would have died.

Today, we know the potential danger of the coronary. But we know, too, that it does not invariably kill—and we are learning how to make it less dangerous.

Progress has been slow but meaningful. Many of the factors contributing to coronary atherosclerosis, the process responsible for narrowing coronary arteries, are being identified. More and more clearly, research is indicating that certain changes of habit, including diet and the pace of life, may reduce the likelihood of a coronary heart attack.

The coronary heart attack itself is better understood. It is now known that many deaths in the past occurred although the heart muscle itself was still relatively healthy—too good to die. The deaths were the result of temporary rhythm disturbances. Today it has become possible to prevent and correct many such disturbances.

As lives are being saved, invalidism is also being reduced. Once upon a heart attack, the physician would say to his patient: "You've had a heart attack; you're going to have to take it easy." An understandably anxious wife might guard her husband from all activity to be sure he did just what the doctor ordered. Very often, a heart attack, even a relatively mild one, was automatically followed by retirement—and fear, depression and bewilderment.

This need no longer happen. The heart is strong—even after a coronary. Well-ordered activity can often keep it strong and make it even stronger.

Even insurance companies, conservative when it comes to assuming risks, are changing their practices. Fifteen years ago a patient with heart trouble could not buy life insurance anywhere. Now this no longer holds. He may buy insurance at extra cost several years after a coronary attack and in ten to fifteen years may pay rates which are practically normal.

Insurance companies are also taking an increasingly optimistic view of patients with repaired congenital defects. In some cases, after a waiting period of one to four years, such patients may obtain insurance at standard rates, and it seems likely that more and more of them will be able to do so in the future.

We still have a long way to go. But we have come far in our

understanding of the heart, its strengths and weaknesses, and how to use its strengths to help overcome its ills and even prevent many of them.

We are at a point now where the more information people have —healthy people, heart patients, families of heart patients—the greater the chance for medicine to win the battle of the heart. This book has been written with the purpose of providing that information.

The book starts with a description of the normal functioning of the heart and then goes into the symptoms that may be related to heart problems. It deals with congenital heart defects, rheumatic heart disease, heart infections of various types. High blood pressure and congestive heart failure are treated in special chapters, as is the question of pregnancy and heart disease.

There are six chapters on the many different aspects of coronary heart disease: the meaning of angina pectoris in relation to heart attack, what happens in an actual heart attack, what happens after one, the personal experience of one of the authors, the need for action when you suspect an attack, and the need for care to try to prevent one.

A special chapter covers the promising new surgical techniques that have been developed to revitalize the heart. Other chapters discuss pacemakers and other electronic helps for the heart, the drugs used to combat heart problems and the present status and likely future of both heart transplants and artificial hearts.

And the book ends as optimistically as it begins—with a discussion of how the many people who mistakenly believe they have heart disease can be freed of needless anxiety.

In the Appendix, we present something we believe to be of great practical value: the American Heart Association's fat-controlled, low-cholesterol meal plan. Coupled with other measures we suggest, we think it can contribute significantly to combating coronary heart disease and heart attacks.

Finally, we have included a dictionary of heart terms.

Our hope is that if you are a heart patient, or if a member of your family is, this book will supplement your doctor's explanations and answer the questions that occur to you from time to time.

We trust that this book will also serve in other ways: as a reference work for the healthy; as a source of information about the symptoms that sometimes occur in everyday life, and when to seek medical advice about them; and, not least, as a practical guide to everyday measures that may help prevent or retard the development of heart disease.

[1]

The Normal Heart

When fully grown, the human heart is only slightly larger than your clenched fist and weighs less than a pound. It roughly resembles a valentine heart in shape—or, somewhat more closely, a ripe eggplant. It is located in the front part of the chest, under the breastbone in the center, with its apex pointed to the left. It is encased in a slippery membrane called the pericardium, which allows it to move freely while keeping it in position.

The heart is a hollow organ (see Figure 1). Its wall is made up of thick muscle called the myocardium. Inside are four hollow chambers, two on the right side of the heart and two on the left. The top chamber on each side is the atrium or receiving chamber; the bottom chamber is the ventricle or pumping chamber. A solid partition of muscle called the septum separates the right atrium and ventricle from the left ones, so that the heart functions as two separate pumps, side by side.

The right side of the heart sends blood that has circulated throughout the body into the lungs to be freshened with oxygen; the left side sends the blood freshened in the lungs back through the body again.

1

This, step by step, is the way the heart works (see Figure 2):

1. After blood has circulated through the body and given up its oxygen, it returns to the heart, entering the right atrium through two great veins, the venae cavae.

2. As the atrium fills, it contracts to pass the blood through the tricuspid valve into the right ventricle.

3. A contraction of the right ventricle propels the blood into the pulmonary artery, which, through branches, carries it to both lungs.

4. Within the lungs, the blood moves into progressively smaller vessels until it reaches the capillaries, each of which has a diameter of about 1/2500 of an inch. In the capillaries, blood cells move in single file and, one by one, give up the carbon dioxide they have collected in the body and receive a fresh supply of oxygen.

5. From the lungs, the freshened blood moves through the four pulmonary veins into the left atrium. As the atrium fills, it contracts to send the blood through the mitral valve into the left ventricle below.

6. With a strong contraction, the left ventricle pumps the blood into the aorta, the body's great trunkline artery, whose diameter is about that of a garden hose. From the aorta, many arteries branch off to carry blood to all areas of the body. The blood, after making the circuit, giving up its oxygen and picking up carbon dioxide, returns to the heart.

The two sides of the heart work in concert; that is, while the right atrium is receiving used blood from the body, the left atrium is receiving fresh blood from the lungs. Both atria contract to send the blood to the ventricles simultaneously. Both atria pause momentarily as the two ventricles contract simultaneously, and the ventricles, in turn, pause while the atria contract.

As the ventricles begin to contract, the tricuspid and mitral valves close to prevent blood from backing up into the atria. After each contraction, two other valves (the pulmonary at the entrance to the pulmonary artery and the aortic at the entrance to the aorta) close to prevent blood from returning to the ventricles.

If you put your ear to someone's chest, over the heart, you can hear a set of sounds: *lubb-dup, lubb-dup, lubb-dup.* The *lubb* is

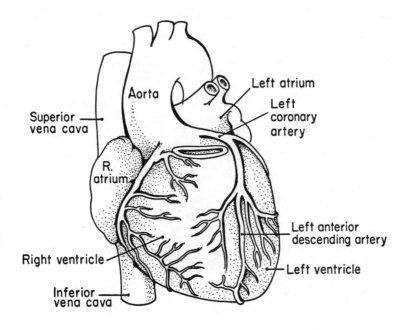

Figure 1. The coronary vessels that supply blood to the heart muscle. They are located on the surface of the heart and originate from the aorta.

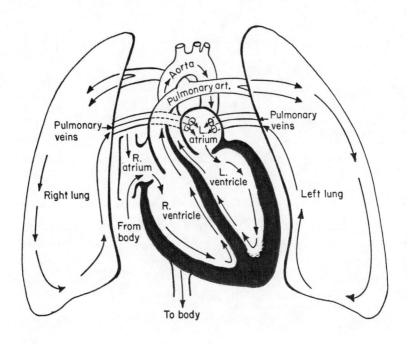

Figure 2. The inside of the heart, showing flow of blood from the head and body to the right atrium, then into the right ventricle and pulmonary artery to the lungs. The blood from the lungs is returned to the left atrium and then to the left ventricle and aorta. From here, blood flows to every organ of the body.

the sound of the closing of the tricuspid and mitral valves; the *dup* is the sound of the closing of the pulmonary and aortic valves.

THE HEART CONTROL MECHANISMS

The normal rate of heartbeat is about seventy to seventy-five a minute. With each beat or contraction, the heart forces about half a cup of blood out to the body so that, in a twenty-four-hour period, it pumps more than 2,600 gallons. When an increased flow of blood is needed, the beat speeds up to as much as twice the normal rate. At the same time, the heart contracts more completely to eject more blood with each beat.

Under normal resting conditions, the ventricles need pump out only about half the blood they contain, but when the need for blood is greater, the ventricles can pump out their total content. Thus, when you exercise, your heart can greatly increase blood flow.

The heart is responsive to increased demand for blood at other times also. For example, during a feverish illness, blood vessels dilate, and the heart pumps more blood to fill them. If an illness involves infection, the extra blood carries with it more white blood cells to help combat the infectious organisms.

A remarkable set of control mechanisms keeps the heart rate suited to the body needs. In the brain is a remote-control heart-rate center which receives nerve signals produced by various phenomena: circulatory-system changes, emotional disturbances, reactions to sights, sounds and other sensory perceptions. The brain center responds by signaling the heart to slow down or speed up.

These signals go to the heart's pacemaker, an area of special tissue in the right atrium which, in effect, sets the rate for the rest of the heart. Tiny electrical signals from the pacemaker spark the atrial muscles to force blood into the ventricles and spark the ventricle muscles to propel the blood out to lungs and body.

Consider, for example, what happens when you start running. As your leg muscles become active, they squeeze leg veins and, by doing so, they speed the return of blood from the legs to the heart via the inferior vena cava. The vena cava stretches to accommodate the increased blood flow, and this very stretching sends a signal to the brain center. The center then signals the pacemaker to fire more rapidly and speed the pumping rhythm of the heart to satisfy your increased need for oxygen as you run.

The heart's own arteries (Figure 1)

Like all other body tissues, the heart muscle itself must have oxygen replenishment and waste removal. A special coronary circulation system takes care of this.

The system begins at the aorta. Near the point where this great vessel emerges from the heart, two coronary arteries branch from it. Each has a diameter about the size of a large knitting needle or a thin pencil. The right coronary supplies mainly the right and back sides of the ventricle areas. The left coronary supplies mainly the left side, part of the front and the back of the heart muscle. Each artery also branches to areas served by the other. (The left coronary quickly divides into two major divisions, which is why it is sometimes said that there are three main arteries that nourish the heart.) The coronary system also includes veins that carry used blood into the right atrium for freshening.

As the heart adapts to body demands, so the coronary circulation adapts to the heart's needs.

The coronary arteries take a required amount of blood from the aorta. When the heart works harder, beating more often and more powerfully, it requires more nourishment, and the coronary circulation accommodates by taking more blood from the aorta.

The coronary arteries have three layers. The middle one contains muscular and elastic tissues that can contract to diminish the artery diameter when relatively little blood is flowing through, and can expand to accommodate greatly increased flow.

The coronary circulation also has extra capillaries which bring more blood to the heart muscle when you exert yourself vigorously. These same capillaries serve as "spares": if some of the regular blood channels for the heart become diseased and no longer function effectively, the capillaries go into regular use as vital substitute pathways.

Since, in addition, many heart areas have blood supplied by both the left and right coronary arteries, if one entire artery should become diseased and narrowed, the other may be able to supply sufficient blood to enable the heart to go on functioning.

So the heart is truly a remarkable pump. It is more efficient than any machine of any kind yet devised by man. It produces so much energy that if its lifetime output could be concentrated into one burst of power it could lift a battleship several feet out of the water.

But it is, of course, subject to disorders. When something goes wrong, how does a doctor determine what it is?

[2]

The Meaning of Symptoms

In recent years, the press, radio and television have contributed materially to the health education of the general public, particularly in regard to the prevention and treatment of various diseases.

But advances in diagnosis are not so well known. The very process of reaching a diagnosis seems mysterious to most people. When it comes to heart disease, there is a great deal of confusion about the meaning of various symptoms, the importance of steps in the examination of the patient and the interrelation of the two.

How does a doctor test for heart disorders? First of all, by taking the patient's history. An accurate, relevant history is an essential tool of medicine. Not infrequently, a complete diagnosis can be reached on the basis of the history alone. Even when this is not possible, a good history can reduce the number of diagnostic possibilities.

The purpose of history-taking is to obtain an accurate description of the patient's feelings and essential discomforts.

You may have noticed that your physician always tries to avoid asking you a leading question. For example, he does not say:

8

"Did you have a squeezing discomfort in the front part of your chest?" Instead, he asks several other questions: "Did you have pain?" "Where was it located?" "What did it feel like?" He waits for the answer to each before asking the next. The answers to the three questions may indeed reveal that there was pain in the front part of the chest and that the chest felt as if it were being squeezed, but the information has come from you without any prompting.

It is important for you as the patient to communicate freely and fully if you are to get the maximum benefit from the examination. Withholding any information from the doctor because you feel that it may not be pertinent can be a disservice to yourself. Answer all his questions, however irrelevant they may seem. And be as precise as you possibly can when you describe how you feel.

People differ in their sensitivity to discomfort and their ability to describe the nature of their symptoms. Some people are relatively insensitive to pain; some have difficulty in localizing pain; others have trouble indicating the character, duration or severity of a symptom. A physician recognizes such differences among patients and makes proper allowances for them.

The symptoms of heart disease vary greatly, depending on the nature and severity of the disorder and how it disturbs the circulation. (In fact, almost any type of heart disorder can be present without producing any symptoms whatever.) It is rare that an individual, on the basis of one or more symptoms, can establish for himself that heart disease is present.

SYMPTOMS AS CLUES

But symptoms are helpful clues. They indicate that something may be wrong. So we urge you to heed them, to make use of them as possible warnings, but *not* to make assumptions about what they mean—assumptions that may lead you to neglect a serious disorder or to fear a disorder you do not have.

We could cite many examples of misinterpretation of symptoms by patients. A classic one is thinking that one's headaches stem from extreme high blood pressure: most forms of high blood pressure do not produce headache. Often patients with shortness of breath believe that they have a heart condition, when theirs is actually a case of deep, sighing respiration brought about by tension and nervousness. And people often interpret palpitations —an extra heartbeat or two—as an indication of serious heart disorder, when in fact they may be entirely innocuous and normal.

Fatigue

Fatigue is a common complaint in all forms of heart disease. When a heart disorder leads to inadequate blood circulation, waste products—mainly lactic acid—accumulate in muscles throughout the body and irritate nerve endings, producing the sensation of fatigue. The heart condition need not be a serious one to cause fatigue.

But fatigue is a common complaint in many other types of illness. It usually develops the first thing in the morning with patients who have emotional disturbances, reflecting their reluctance to face the difficulties of the day. In most heart cases, on the contrary, fatigue does not occur in early-morning hours if the patient has had a reasonable amount of rest and sleep.

Cardiac fatigue varies from a mild form to a seriously incapacitating one. If mild, it may not be recognized as a disability because the patient often adjusts activities to avoid the sensation of tiredness. In many instances, patients who have recovered from heart disease report that they did not really understand the magnitude of their fatigue until after their recovery, when they were able to compare it with their newfound sense of well-being.

In its more serious form, fatigue may appear as a disability or ache, distributed over the entire body, that makes the patient feel sick, and that is not completely eliminated even by a long period of rest.

The important points to keep in mind about fatigue as a possible symptom of heart trouble are:

1. It varies greatly in magnitude.

2. It is present in other forms of disease—and so every fatigued person does not necessarily have heart disease.

3. In many cases patients automatically, unconsciously, adjust their physical output to avoid fatigue—and hence many people with heart trouble are not so aware of the symptom as they should be.

Pain

Pain occurs with many types of heart disease. The most common is that of coronary heart disease, in which inadequate blood flow to the heart muscle produces discomfort in the chest.

Pain is also produced by congenital heart disease and may be present in rheumatic heart disease. It is encountered, too, when the covering of the heart, the pericardium, becomes inflamed. It may occur when there is an irregular heart action—and sometimes even with normal increases in heart rate.

Heart-related pain is generally located in the chest area either immediately over the left breast or in the center, beneath the breast bone (sternum).

The way in which the pain begins, its character and its duration may help the physician to determine its probable cause. But often this is not a simple matter.

The pain associated with coronary heart disease is called angina pectoris (see Chapter 9). It is often described as an oppressive sensation in the center of the chest. At times, patients report it to be a burning, bandlike, or squeezing discomfort. Characteristically, it is brief in duration and closely related to physical effort, often disappearing within two or three minutes after the patient stops the effort. Even when the pain is not intense, it is accompanied by a feeling of impending disaster which is compelling enough to force the person to stop or slow down any activity. The pain may radiate to the shoulders and down both arms, or into the neck or jaws and through to the back. It is more likely to radiate to the left than to the right. (Only about 10 percent of patients experience pain radiation to the right shoulder and arm.)

The pain associated with high blood pressure in the pulmonary, or lung, circuit closely resembles that of coronary heart disease.

The pain of pericardial inflammation is distinctive: it is sharp, cutting, limited to the left side of the chest and clearly related to and aggravated by deep breathing. There are distinguishing features, too, for the pain associated with irregular heart action: the discomfort is dull, persistent, not related to activity and likely to be localized over the left breast and in the center of the chest.

In brief:

1. Chest pain may be produced by a number of heart disorders, but nonheart conditions, too, may cause pain in the chest area.

2. Of all causes of heart-related chest pain, coronary heart disease is the most common and serious.

3. The chest pain of coronary heart disease is generally triggered by stress, either physical or emotional, and usually disappears as soon as the stress is ended.

4. This sort of chest pain (angina pectoris) is apt to be transmitted to other body areas, most commonly the left upper and lower arm, the left fingertips, the right shoulder and upper arm, the base of the throat, the jaws and/or the neck. On rare occasions, it affects the ear lobes.

5. Serious cardiac pain commonly brings with it a sense of impending disaster, and so the patient is not likely to tolerate it for long periods without seeking medical aid. Hence, any chest pain that is endured for hours at a time, tends to be vague and does not compel the patient to seek medical help is probably not caused by a heart condition.

Shortness of Breath (Dyspnea)

Shortness of breath, or labored breathing, often accompanies heart disease. It arises because the pumping power of the heart has been reduced, so blood accumulates in lung vessels, which then swell and compress air spaces in the lungs.

The degree of breathlessness can vary greatly, causing mild discomfort during active exercise or labored breathing even at rest.

But breathlessness rarely develops suddenly in a heart patient. It starts generally with breathing difficulty during physical effort. Such difficulty is, of course, common to many adults who are simply not in good physical condition. But the breathlessness of the heart patient during exercise is generally greater in magnitude and will gradually occur with less and less effort. Eventually, the patient may be breathless when at rest or even while asleep. In the latter case, he may need to prop his head up with pillows to avoid a feeling of suffocation.

Breathlessness which develops sporadically with exercise or during periods of rest is called paroxysmal dyspnea. The type which develops at night, even during sleep, is called nocturnal dyspnea. Nocturnal dyspnea indicates a more serious defect in heart function.

Breathlessness may result from nonheart disorders, particularly those involving the lungs. Again, some people may confuse deep, sighing respirations stemming from emotional problems with breathlessness. The deep sighs are characterized by lengthy inspiration, breathing in. In breathlessness, inspiration and expiration are generally of equal duration and the rate is usually rapid.

Swelling of the Extremities (Edema)

When the heart does not pump effectively, blood flow to the kidneys is impaired. The kidneys then do not do a thorough job of eliminating salt and water. As a result, the body tissues, particularly in the extremities, tend to become swollen with fluid.

But fluid accumulation (edema) occurs in many nonheart conditions. It is common in people who have poor circulation in their leg veins—often manifested by varicose veins or clots within the vein system. In women, a certain amount of edema may occur from salt and water retention produced by hormonal changes during the menstrual cycle. Leg swelling is not uncommon in kidney disease and in certain nutritional disorders.

While edema generally indicates an organic disease process, it does not necessarily mean a serious process.

A considerable quantity of fluid must accumulate in the tissue spaces before it becomes noticeable. Hence, edema—when it is heart-caused—is usually not among the first signs of the condition.

Edema associated with a heart problem usually tends to appear late in the day. Only when the heart condition is advanced is it observed in the early morning before any activity has taken place.

When there is significant edema, finger pressure on the lower part of the ankles and the shinbone leaves a depression which lasts for several minutes. This is called pitting edema. When a heart condition worsens, edema may also be noticed in the soft tissues of the upper part of the legs—and sometimes may even become severe enough to involve the genital organs and lower part of the back.

Palpitation

Palpitation means an abnormal rate or rhythm of the heart. Under normal circumstances, we are not conscious of the rate or rhythm of the heartbeat. When, after exercise, the heartbeat speeds up, we are aware of a pounding sensation in the chest. But it disappears so quickly after exercise and is so obviously related to the exercise that it is seldom mistaken for an abnormality.

Many people have experienced the sensation of having their heart seem to skip a beat. Some are aware at times of an extra-powerful beat of the heart. Both sensations are part of the same phenomenon: A premature electrical stimulus to the heart muscle makes it contract too early. The early contraction occurs when the heart has not filled with blood, and so a smaller amount than usual is pumped out. After such an early beat, there is a longer-than-usual pause while the heart fills up with a greater amount of blood to make up for the earlier shortage. The first heartbeat after the pause therefore ejects an unusually large amount of blood into the aorta, producing a large pulsation which becomes noticeable. Such a simple palpitation may occur in almost any normal individual.

Abnormalities of heart rate and rhythm may be the result of disorders elsewhere in the body. For example, hyperthyroidism, a condition in which the thyroid gland is overactive and produces excessive secretions of thyroid hormone, may overstimulate the whole body and greatly increase the heart rate, and may also cause rapid bursts of an abnormal rhythm known as atrial fibrillation.

But there are many other types of rhythm abnormalities which may be associated with heart disease.

It is helpful to the physician if a patient who complains of palpitations can report as clearly as possible not only his impression of the abnormality but also the conditions under which it appears.

Abnormalities of rate and rhythm can usually be treated effectively. Some are related to excessive smoking or excessive intake of coffee (or, occasionally, alcohol). When an overactive thyroid is the cause, proper diagnosis and treatment for the thyroid condition can stop the palpitations as well as produce a general improvement in health. And there are medications to control and prevent recurrences of heart-related rate and rhythm abnormalities.

Fainting (Syncope)

Fainting, or syncope, may be the result of a heart disorder, but there are many other possible causes.

In a common faint, an emotional disturbance such as fear or anxiety affects the control center that regulates the size of blood vessels; many vessels become dilated and, with such enlargement, blood pressure falls; the blood does not therefore have enough push behind it to overcome the force of gravity and reach the height of the brain, and so fainting takes place. But spontaneous recovery is inevitable, because the unconscious state wipes out the stimulus of fear, anxiety or other emotion—while the horizontal position of the patient helps restore blood flow to the brain.

Fainting may also be produced by excessive loss of blood, or by extreme pain which reduces blood pressure to very low levels. Sometimes fainting may be caused by drugs which lower blood pressure excessively.

Fainting associated with heart disease occurs when the heart fails to maintain adequate blood flow to the brain. This may be because of momentary heart stoppage, abnormal heart rhythm, heart-valve disease or embolism—the formation of a blood clot which lodges in and blocks a lung or brain blood vessel.

But sudden fainting is rarely the first indication of heart disease. It is more likely to occur in the patient not known to have a heart problem.

Blood-Spitting (Hemoptysis)

Blood-spitting, or hemoptysis, sometimes represents a relatively unimportant problem. It may even be caused by coughing during a common cold. But since it may indicate a significant disorder, heart or nonheart, it should be reported immediately to a physician.

Hemoptysis usually occurs when lung tissue is inundated with blood—perhaps because the mitral valve has become obstructed as the result of rheumatic heart disease, or because the left ventricle of the heart is not functioning well as a result of high blood pressure, coronary heart disease or aortic-valve disease.

Blood-spitting may also occur when a blood clot passes to a lung from somewhere else in the body, or when there is a lung infection or tumor.

Cough

The causes of a cough range from common respiratory infections to lung tumors. When coughing is associated with heart disease, it is usually the result of the lung or bronchial (airway) tissue's filling with fluid because of impaired circulation. In some cases, a cough may be produced by the pressure of a greatly enlarged heart chamber on a bronchial tube or airway.

A cardiac cough is generally described as a chronic, unyielding annoyance. It tends to be aggravated after exercise. It may also be aggravated when a patient is lying down on his back. At first a cardiac cough may be dry, but later there may be large amounts of frothy sputum, often blood-tinged.

Insomnia

Many heart patients complain that they have difficulty sleeping. Sleep may be disturbed by actual pain, by irregular heart rate or rhythm, or by cough or breathlessness. In some cases sleep may be disturbed by inadequate blood flow to the brain resulting from poor heart-muscle contraction.

Because there are many reasons for insomnia completely unrelated to the heart, it should never be assumed that a sleeping problem indicates a cardiac condition.

Sexual Impotence

Ordinarily, loss of sexual ability stems from psychological disturbances. Impotence in heart patients may reflect psychological difficulties or may be the result of heart disturbances precipitated by the effort involved.

Sex play and the sex act increase the work of the heart. In patients with hypertensive heart disease, the increased effort may cause breathlessness; patients with coronary heart disease may suffer breathlessness, chest pain or abnormal heart rhythms; and patients with rheumatic heart disease may also be breathless and have abnormal heart rhythms. In patients with aortic-valve disease, sexual activity may lead to fainting.

Usually, impotence based on such symptoms does not develop except in advanced forms of heart disease. When it occurs in patients who are not seriously incapacitated, psychological rather than organic factors may be responsible.

Indigestion

Abdominal discomfort may be associated with heart disease. Not uncommonly, the angina of coronary heart disease is misinterpreted as indigestion. Abdominal pain may result from distention of the liver caused by inadequate heart pumping and circulation.

Gastrointestinal symptoms, including loss of appetite, belching, and a sense of fullness, may occur in coronary heart disease, some forms of congenital heart disease and hypertensive heart disease. But it must be remembered that such symptoms are common to many other conditions which have nothing to do with the heart.

Vertigo (Dizziness)

Dizziness is occasionally a symptom of heart disease, the result of a momentary abnormal rhythm which briefly reduces the output of the heart—not enough to cause fainting but enough to disturb the balancing centers in the middle ear and brain.

But it must be emphasized that dizziness occurs with many nonheart conditions—and frequently occurs when there is no significant disease problem at all.

THE PHYSICIAN'S FINDINGS

But the physician does not limit himself to learning the patient's symptoms. He is also making findings himself. Even as he is taking the case history, the physician is making a preliminary general inspection of the patient. He is observing his body build and appearance, the color of his skin, his breathing rate, his attitude and any indications of pain or anxiety.

The Pulse

The physician often begins the physical examination by taking the patient's pulse. The pulse rate is usually the same as the heart rate, but with a very rapid or irregular heart rate the pulse may be slower.

The normal pulse rate generally ranges from sixty to eighty beats a minute, with seventy-two as the average. Values below sixty in health are unusual, but values above eighty may occur in some healthy people, for the pulse rate varies considerably between different people and in the same person at different times.

Exercise and emotional stress increase the pulse rate. So does fever. The rate also increases when blood pressure is elevated and when hyperthyroidism is present. And an increased rate does occur with some forms of heart disease: when, for example, the heart is said to be in congestive failure, and also at times when there is disease of the pericardium, the sac that envelops the heart.

On the other hand, the pulse rate *slows* in some heart disorders, as well as in hypothyroidism (underfunctioning of the thyroid gland).

The physician can gain much information about the functioning of the heart from various characteristics of the pulse: its strength, rate and rhythm—whether there are alternations of large and small pulses.

There are pulsations in the veins, too, less vigorous than those in the arteries and best seen in the jugular veins in the neck. Observation of the characteristics of these pulsations can help determine whether there are structural defects in some of the heart valves or other abnormalities.

Arms, Legs and Peripheral Circulation

The physician examines the arms, legs and, in fact, much of the body to evaluate the peripheral circulation—that is, how blood is transported to the extremities and throughout the body.

When the skin is pale and cold, the reason is usually that small blood vessels of the skin have contracted—as they will quite normally in response to environmental temperature. But they may also contract when the heart does not pump normally because of various heart problems.

Blueness of the skin and fingernail beds is called cyanosis. There are two types. One, peripheral cyanosis, occurs in exposed areas of the body, and disappears when the areas are warm. The second, central cyanosis, is seen in protected portions of the body, such as the inner surfaces of the lips, and occurs when there is a mixture of oxygen-rich and oxygen-poor blood within the heart as the result of a congenital defect—the "blue baby."

When the skin is unusually warm, it indicates peripheral vasodilation—relaxation and widening of blood vessels of the skin. This occurs as a normal reaction to hot temperatures, but also as the result of a high heart output (such as may be present during pregnancy), increased thyroid-gland function or abnormal communicating channels between arteries and veins. As the blood flow increases, the skin blood vessels dilate to make room for the increased flow.

The physician examines the extremities, especially the legs, for any swelling indicating abnormal fluid accumulation.

He examines the fingers and toes carefully for any "clubbing" —thickening and enlargement of the end portions of the fingers and toes which give them a spatula-like appearance. Clubbing occurs commonly with central cyanosis and therefore suggests the presence of congenital heart disease; or it may sometimes indicate a chronic respiratory ailment. It should be noted, however, that clubbing may be present in some people even though they have no heart or lung disorder; apparently, in them it is a familial characteristic without health significance.

Blood Pressure

Blood-pressure measurement is an important part of the physical examination. The instrument used for it is called a sphygmomanometer.

A cuff attached to the sphygmomanometer is wrapped around the arm above the elbow and inflated until the blood flow is interrupted. Then, with his stethoscope placed lightly over the large artery in the inner area of the elbow, the physician slowly deflates the cuff. As the cuff deflates, he listens for the first pulsations that indicate that blood has begun to flow again. This happens when the pressure of blood in the artery equals the pressure of air in the cuff. This is called systolic pressure, and it indicates the force with which blood is ejected from the heart, the pressure in the artery when the heartbeat occurs. The physician reads the value on the sphygmomanometer dial or meter.

As the cuff deflates further, the initial sharp sounds of blood flow are succeeded by muffled sounds. At this point the physician can determine the pressure *between* heartbeats, called diastolic pressure.

Blood-pressure values are expressed in millimeters of mercury, and a blood-pressure reading consists of two figures: the higher value, the systolic pressure, written first, and the lower value, the diastolic, next. For example: 120/80.

Normal systolic pressure is in the range of 100 to 140. There is comfort in having a systolic pressure with lower rather than higher value. Although it is true that systolic pressures in older people (usually above the age of fifty) tend to be generally higher than in younger people, the pressure elevation that takes place with aging is thought to be more likely the result of loss of flexibility of blood vessels.

The normal diastolic pressure lies in the range of 60 to 90. Diastolic pressure does not normally elevate with aging. Any elevation beyond 90 is considered above normal limits regardless of age.

It is easy for inaccurate blood-pressure readings to be taken. If a patient has rushed to keep an appointment with the physician, or is anxious about the examination and what it may show, or is disturbed for any other reason, the readings may be higher than they would otherwise be. Very often, therefore, the physician takes a second blood pressure at the end of the physical examination to make sure that the first reading is an accurate indication of the patient's usual blood-pressure level.

Usually the patient sits or lies down for a blood-pressure reading, but sometimes the physician has him stand, for he may suspect orthostatic hypotension—a condition in which blood pressure drops sharply when the patient stands. This is most frequent in a patient with high blood pressure who has been receiving drugs to reduce the pressure. Orthostatic hypotension does not always develop with drug treatment—and when it does, it can be overcome by a change in dosage of the drug or by use of an alternative drug or drugs.

Eyes

Often, before examining the heart itself, the physician studies the patient's eyes. By shining a light from an instrument called an ophthalmoscope through the pupils of the eyes, he can view the retina and its blood vessels.

His objective is not to appraise vision but to judge the state of health of blood vessels tinier than any that can be seen readily elsewhere in the body. By viewing these vessels and searching for evidence of hemorrhaging, the physician obtains clues about the presence or absence of artery hardening. In addition, if the patient is found to have high blood pressure, the condition of the tiny vessels provides some indication of how long the elevated pressure may have been present before discovery.

The Heart Itself

The physician begins his examination of the heart with a visual inspection of the chest. Sometimes a deformity in the chest develops because of a curvature of the spine. And the deformity may displace the heart enough to create murmurs or other seemingly abnormal heart sounds. On the other hand, a bulge in the front chest wall may occur when there is a significant congenital defect of the heart that has led to overdevelopment of the right pumping chamber. So chest inspection may provide valuable clues.

After inspecting the chest, the physician palpates it—feels with sensitive, trained fingers. A pulsation known as the apex beat usually occurs in the space between the fifth and sixth ribs. Normally it is weak. An exaggeration of the apex beat may indicate a heart problem—most often, an increase in the size of the left pumping chamber. The exaggerated beat is easily felt by the physician's palpating hand. Sometimes the physician feels a "thrill" while palpating—a vibratory sensation which may be indicative of a heart problem.

Next the physician listens to the heart through his stethoscope. Auscultation, the medical term for this, provides much valuable information. The contracting heart produces "first" and "second" sounds. The *lubb* that occurs as the mitral and tricuspid valves close is the first sound. The *dup* produced by the closing of the pulmonary and aortic valves is the second sound. Any abnormal changes in these sounds may be helpful in diagnosis.

Auscultation also makes it possible to detect murmurs. Murmurs are noises—vibrations of varying frequency, intensity, quality and duration—which may be produced by structural abnormalities in the heart or by peculiarities in the way blood flows through the chambers of the heart.

Knowing when a murmur occurs—its precise time in the operating cycle of the heart—and also its intensity and general characteristics, the physician is often able to identify the structural defect or blood-transport fault which produces it.

But there are many *innocent* murmurs, too. These may be produced by slight quirks in the way blood flows and have no real significance because they do not indicate heart disease. Innocent murmurs generally are recognized by their location (most are heard on the chest at the left of the breastbone) and by changes in their intensity and quality produced by simple changes in posture and breathing.

Special Examinations

X Rays. Many X-ray methods are available today for use in diagnosing heart conditions:

Teleradiography is a routine method of x-raying the chest and providing a film record of the shape and size of the heart.

Fluoroscopy is a routine method which does not provide a film but has the advantage of allowing the physician to see the heart at work. By changing the patient's position, the physician can observe not only the heart but the diaphragm, lungs and other structures in various perspectives.

Angiocardiography is a method by which the heart chambers, blood vessels and course of blood flow can be seen with the aid of a contrast material. With the development of surgical procedures capable of correcting many heart defects, angiocardiography has proved to be invaluable and is being used with greater frequency.

It is usually carried out in a hospital. The patient is given local anesthesia and a small incision is made into a blood vessel in an area such as the crease of the elbow. Then a long, thin, flexible tube called a catheter is placed in the blood vessel. Following its course on a fluoroscope screen with the aid of a special image intensifier, the physician maneuvers the catheter up through the vessel and into the heart. The patient feels nothing while this is going on.

Then a harmless contrast material is injected into the catheter and soon reaches the heart. X-ray films taken at intervals provide a clear picture of great value. In addition to revealing heart and blood-vessel structure, they show heart activity, the motion of the heart valves, the flow of blood. They are being used increasingly to help in diagnosing congenital heart disorders and many other types of heart conditions. They are also being used to examine the coronary arteries and to determine whether surgery can be helpful for patients with coronary heart disease. This procedure is called *coronary arteriography*.

Cardiac Catheterization.   This is another important diagnostic aid involving the introduction of a catheter into the heart. Through the catheter, precise measurements are made of pressure and flows within the chambers of the heart and of other factors which help the physician assess the working of the heart and major blood vessels in fine detail. The angiocardiography and the cardiac catheterization can be carried out in the same session, one following the other.

Electrocardiography. The electrocardiograph is frequently used to measure the electrical forces generated by the heart.

Each cell in the heart muscle is virtually a microscopic battery which discharges a current when active, then recharges itself during rest. The current discharge begins in an area on the right side of the heart—the pacemaker—and spreads almost instantaneously over the entire heart along definite pathways and then over the body and to the skin. Electrodes placed on the skin pick up these signals, and the electrocardiograph amplifies them and produces a record, the electrocardiogram, on a moving strip of graph paper.

The record takes the form of a series of waves designated by the letters P, Q, R, S, T and U. Changes in the various waves indicate the rhythm and rate of heart action, the time it takes for the electrical impulse to spread from pacemaker to entire heart, the functional capacity of the fibers that transmit the electrical impulse, and any injury or destruction of heart muscle.

The electrocardiogram is a diagnostic aid, but only that. It provides useful information, but the information must be interpreted carefully and with regard to findings the physician makes through other means. The electrocardiogram does not identify causes of abnormalities, nor does it necessarily predict the likelihood of a heart problem developing at some time in the future. It is possible to have a serious heart disease which does not indicate its presence by electrocardiographic abnormalities, and it is possible to have electrocardiographic abnormalities when there is no serious heart problem.

Phonocardiography. This is a technique of recording heart sounds. Rarely does a phonocardiogram show up any sounds that the physician cannot hear through his stethoscope. It merely records them in graphic form. Occasionally, however, it may be needed to define more clearly the sounds heard through the stethoscope.

Ultrasound Cardiography, or Echocardiography. This is a method of recording the echoes of ultrasonic waves—very-high-frequency sound waves beyond the range of hearing—when these waves are made to strike heart areas by placing a high-frequency generator on the chest wall. The principle is the same as that used in radar recognition of airplanes and submarines. The procedure is simple, no more troublesome for the patient than electrocardiography. The technique is helpful in showing up abnormalities of heart valves, especially of the mitral valve; abnormal fluid in the pericardium; abnormal thickening of the heart muscle itself; and any abnormal growth or tumor within a heart chamber.

As you can see, diagnosis of heart disease is not arrived at instantly and on the basis of impressions only. It calls for careful study to elicit as accurate a picture as possible of the patient's symptoms, then further study to determine what really accounts for the symptoms: whether they stem from a heart problem or from something entirely different; and if they do come from the heart, what the problem is.

You cannot expect to be able to determine for yourself whether or not you have heart disease. And that is not simply because you do not have the technical training or all of the diagnostic aids. The fact is that no sensible physician would ever try to determine whether he himself has heart trouble or how serious it might be. He would consult another physician, because he would realize that he is too emotionally involved with his problem to be able to come to a clear, level-headed decision about it.

What we hoped to do in this chapter was to give you an awareness of what goes into making a diagnosis of heart disease, so that you can approach your medical examinations more knowledgeably and be better able to cooperate in them and so that if you become aware of a new symptom, you will recognize the wisdom of discussing it with your physician.

[3]

Congenital Defects: Heart Problems Children Are Born With

Each year in the United States 30,000 to 40,000 babies are born with heart defects. But today, for most of this relatively small but precious group of children, the outlook is excellent. They can benefit from remarkable advances in diagnosis, medical treatment and corrective surgery. For the picture for children with congenital heart defects has changed much and quickly.

One of the first successful attempts to correct a congenital, or inborn, defect was made in 1939 when Dr. Robert Gross, of Harvard Medical School, performed an operation on a seven-year-old girl who had a patent ductus arteriosus, one of the defects we will discuss in this chapter. It was only five years later that Drs. Alfred Blalock and Helen Taussig of Johns Hopkins Hospital in Baltimore devised an operation to help the "blue baby," the victim of a combination of four heart defects.

To see a child who was once deep blue and virtually unable to walk across a room turn a healthy pink after an operation and, within weeks, run through hospital corridors—this is an experience as rewarding for physicians as for parents.

27

Not all heart defects lend themselves readily to surgery, but research is constantly paving the way for more of them to be so treated when necessary.

And not all congenital heart defects require surgery. Some are so mild that, with effective medical care now available, the patient can live a virtually normal life without an operation.

WHAT CAUSES CONGENITAL DEFECTS?

Every doctor wishes he knew the answer, but it is not yet entirely clear.

If a mother has German measles during the first three months of her pregnancy, the normal development of her baby's heart may be affected. German measles is a virus disease, and the possibility that other virus diseases early in pregnancy may be responsible for at least some congenital heart defects is under study.

The role of heredity is still uncertain and is being actively studied. While more than one child in a family may have a congenital heart defect, such cases are rare. It has been estimated that parents who have one child born with a heart defect run a risk no greater than one in fifty of having a second child with a heart defect.

Can drugs taken during pregnancy lead to malformation of the baby's heart? This, too, is unsettled. In animal studies, some substances have been found to cause malformations, but whether this may hold true in humans is not yet known.

We do not yet have precise knowledge of the influence of the mother's diet on all aspects of her baby's prenatal development. It is known, however, that the mother's own health depends on good nutrition, and that a healthy mother is more likely to give birth to a healthy baby than an unhealthy mother is.

TYPES AND DEGREES OF DEFECTS

There are many kinds of congenital heart defects. A defect may be within the heart itself or outside the heart in a nearby major blood vessel. For example, there may be a hole in the wall, or septum, separating two chambers of the heart; or there may be a connection between two major blood vessels where there should be none; or there may be a narrowing of a valve or a blood vessel so that blood flow is hampered. Sometimes there are combinations of several defects. And there are all degrees of defects, with the mildest having virtually no effect on the functioning of the heart.

Because it is of concern to so many parents, we would like to emphasize here that a congenital defect, mild or severe, does not cause mental retardation. When a child with a heart defect is also mentally defective, this means that he was born with two separate defects, not that the heart problem affected the brain. It may happen that a normally intelligent child, tiring easily because of a heart defect, does not do as well as he could in school; but after the defect is corrected, he can be expected to catch up.

While there are many possible congenital defects, some are extremely rare. The following eight account for more than 90 percent of the total:

Patent ductus arteriosus
Coarctation of the aorta
Atrial septal defect
Ventricular septal defect
Pulmonary stenosis
Aortic stenosis
Tetralogy of Fallot
Transposition of great vessels

Patent Ductus Arteriosus

Every infant at birth has a patent ductus arteriosus—a duct or channel that conducts blood between the pulmonary artery and the aorta. The channel is needed before but not after birth.

Before birth, the lungs do not function (the mother's circulation takes care of freshening the baby's blood), and the ductus arteriosus transports blood between the pulmonary artery and the aorta, bypassing the lungs. Before birth, then, the ductus is patent or open. After birth, the lungs do function, the pulmonary artery can take blood from the right side of the heart to the lungs for freshening with oxygen, and the aorta can then carry fresh blood from the left side of the heart to the rest of the body. And so normally, within a few weeks after birth, the ductus arteriosus, no longer needed, closes off and, in time, shrivels up.

If the ductus fails to close, remains patent, some of the fresh, oxygenated blood that flows through the aorta is shunted back into the pulmonary artery and needlessly circulated back to the lungs. In some cases, as much as half of the blood leaving the left ventricle to go to the body—the head, trunk and limbs— may instead go back to the lungs.

In order to maintain adequate circulation for the whole body when so much blood is being returned to the lungs, the heart's efforts must be greatly increased. The heart accommodates to the job, but over an extended period of time it may suffer damage and lose its pumping efficiency. The child's growth may be slowed. And there is risk that infection may arise as bacteria multiply in the ductus—although this, thanks to modern anti-biotics, no longer represents the serious complication it once did.

A child with patent ductus arteriosus may have no symptoms at all or may have blueness of the lower half of the body and clubbing of the toes. In any case, the condition can be detected by the whirring, machinerylike murmur the physician hears through his stethoscope during a physical examination. The murmur is produced by the flow of blood through the open channel. In some children, it may be necessary to confirm the diagnosis with the aid of catheterization (see page 24).

Surgical closure of the ductus corrects the anomaly completely. It was patent ductus arteriosus, as we indicated earlier, which was the first congenital defect to become amenable to surgery.

The operation is relatively simple. Since the duct is located outside the heart, no heart-lung machine or other special equip-ment is needed. The ductus is simply tied off and cut. The correction is permanent. While prompt operation is generally indicated when there is a large flow of blood through the duct, the operation is so safe now that in many medical centers it is performed—to prevent infection—even when the flow is so small that a serious effect on the circulation is not likely.

Within two to three weeks after the operation, a typical patient is thriving, free of murmur, normal in every respect and able to look forward to normal life expectancy.

Coarctation of the Aorta

Like patent ductus arteriosus, this involves a blood vessel near the heart rather than the heart itself. It is a pinching or con-striction (coarctation) of the aorta, the great artery that carries blood from the heart for distribution throughout the body.

The pinching, which may be minor or so great that only a pinpoint channel remains, usually occurs just beyond the point in the aorta at which arteries branch off to carry blood to the head and arms.

Since the narrowing obstructs blood flow, blood pressure in-creases much as water pressure does in a garden hose when you tighten the nozzle. The pressure elevation occurs in the blood vessels of the arms and head before the point of narrowing in the aorta. Long-continued excessive pressure may result, later in life, in damage to the blood vessels in the head and eyes, leading to stroke or visual disturbance. And because the long-continued high pressure causes the heart to work harder in pumping blood into the aorta, the heart may begin to lose effectiveness.

As a rule, a child with coarctation of the aorta has no trouble-some symptoms. Usually, the condition is discovered during a physical examination when blood pressure is found to be high. If a physician finds high blood pressure in the arms of a child during a routine examination, he will take the blood pressure in the child's legs as well; if the child has coarctation of the aorta, the pressure in the legs will be lower than the pressure in the arms.

Again, when surgery is used to correct coarctation, there is no need to go into the heart. The constricted segment is removed and the healthy portions of the aorta are joined. If the section that must be removed is long, a synthetic graft may be placed between the healthy sections.

The operation usually produces a complete cure. After a stay of about two weeks in a hospital, the patient is usually ready to go home in good health.

Atrial Septal Defect

A baby is sometimes born with an abnormal opening in the upper septum, the part of the wall that separates the left and right atria of the heart. This is an atrial septal defect, which allows blood to flow from the left atrium to the right atrium. The amount of blood will depend, of course, on the size of the septal opening. Generally, it is substantial.

The blood from the left atrium has already been to the lungs for freshening. Nevertheless, when the right atrium receives it, it sends it to the right ventricle, which must eject it to the lungs. The right atrium and right ventricle must work harder and thus increase in size. Later in life, the heart may weaken under the extra work and lose the ability to pump efficiently. During childhood, the increased blood flow through the lungs is associated with reduced resistance to respiratory infections, and the child with an atrial septal defect may suffer from repeated chest colds and pneumonia.

At birth, an infant with the defect seldom has any symptoms. With growth and development, a mild tendency to become tired and shortness of breath may appear.

The diagnosis of an atrial septal defect is made on the basis of several findings. A murmur stemming from the increased blood flow through the pulmonary valve can be detected over the base of the heart to the left of the breastbone. X-ray examination of the heart shows some enlargement of the right side, and the pulmonary artery stands out prominently on the X-ray film because of the increased blood flow through it. In addition, there are changes in the electrocardiogram that indicate strain on the right half of the heart

While the diagnosis can be made by an expert physician at this point, the final diagnosis comes after catheterization, which makes it possible to establish clearly not only the presence of the opening in the septum but also its size and the magnitude of the abnormal shunting of blood.

Complete cure can be obtained by surgery. Even in a child in whom an atrial septal defect is causing no serious trouble, surgical correction is advisable to avoid the defect's stressful effects over the years on the right side of the heart. Closing of the hole is best done before the right side becomes irreversibly enlarged. Generally the most suitable time for the operation is when the child is between six and twelve.

The operation is relatively simple because a machine can take over the work of the heart and lungs. (See Chapter 17.) With blood detoured through the heart-lung machine, the heart stays relatively bloodless and the surgeon can open it and close the opening in the septum. If the opening is small, it can be stitched closed. If large, a patch can be used to close it. The closing is permanent.

The operation takes two to three hours. The patient is in the hospital for ten to fourteen days and back in school within four weeks. There are usually no complications after surgery, and the child has a normal life expectancy, especially if the operation is performed before the heart becomes greatly enlarged.

There is another kind of atrial septal defect, called osteum primum. This is an opening in the lower part of the atrial septum, just above the tricuspid and mitral valves, that interferes with the efficient closing of one or the other valve. With this defect, symptoms tend to appear earlier: quick fatigue, shortness of breath and, in some cases, failure to show normal growth and development. The heart is generally larger; the electrocardiogram is more disturbed; and X rays will show a heart even more abnormal than that with the higher atrial septal defect.

Diagnosis of osteum primum can be made by catheterization and by X rays taken after contrast medium is injected. The films show leakage of blood across either the tricuspid or mitral valve.

Osteum primum also is correctable by surgery, but the procedure is more complex than with a simple septal defect. The opening in the septum must be closed and the defective valve repaired. In some instances, when the valve cannot be repaired adequately, a plastic valve is used as a replacement.

Ventricular Septal Defect

Just as some infants are born with an opening between the upper chambers of the heart, some have an abnormal opening between the ventricles, the two lower chambers. This is a ventricular septal defect.

It may be so small in size that no treatment is needed, but with a large defect, blood is shunted from the left ventricle to the right ventricle. The shunting is from left to right because pressure in the left ventricle, which pumps blood to all parts of the body, is naturally higher that the pressure in the right ventricle, which has to pump blood only to the relatively nearby lungs.

As blood is shunted, pressure goes up abnormally in the right ventricle and the increased pressure is transmitted to the lungs, sometimes producing abnormal changes in the blood vessels there.

With a sizable ventricular septal defect, the usual symptoms are labored breathing and fatigue on exertion. Infants under the age of one may have breathing difficulty even at rest. Especially during infancy, there is great susceptibility to prolonged upper-respiratory infection. Children with a large defect are often undersized because the flow of blood to the lungs is greater than the flow to the rest of the body.

Diagnosis rests on much the same procedure as for an atrial septal defect. The stethoscope reveals a murmur, harsh in quality. X-ray examination shows enlargement of the heart and a very prominent pulmonary artery. There are electrocardiographic changes. The exact location of the defect can be determined by catheterization and X-ray studies after injection of contrast medium.

Very small defects may produce loud murmurs and yet give rise to no symptoms; with a small defect, there may be no rise in right heart pressure and no serious lung changes. In some cases, small defects close spontaneously, although it is not known how often this happens. In any event, as we have said, small defects may not require surgery.

When surgery is required, the procedure is much the same as for an atrial septal defect. With the aid of the heart-lung machine, the surgeon can work within the heart, closing the opening by stitching it or, if the opening is too large for that, inserting a patch. The operation takes two to three hours, the patient is home from the hospital in about two weeks and the outlook is usually excellent. The murmur and symptoms disappear, and the patient can expect a normal, healthy life.

In some infants with a large defect, a temporary surgical procedure is required. (Surgeons generally prefer not to do permanent procedures on children less than two or three years old, for the size of the heart and other factors add to the technical difficulties.) The temporary procedure consists of opening the baby's chest and placing a band around the outside of the pulmonary artery. This reduces blood flow to the lung and also increases the pressure in the right side of the heart. The increased pressure helps to reduce the amount of blood shunted into the right ventricle from the left ventricle. The temporary procedure can be lifesaving. When the defect is closed permanently, the band can be removed.

Pulmonary Stenosis

The pulmonary valve regulates the flow of blood from the right ventricle of the heart through the pulmonary artery, which transports the blood to the lungs. But some children are born with a stenosed, or narrowed, pulmonary valve. As a result, the amount of blood going to the lungs is reduced, and body tissues get less than their needed supply of fresh blood. Also, the strain of pumping blood through the narrowed valve may cause the right side of the heart to become enlarged.

Stenosis may occur in the valve itself or in an area very close to the valve. When the stenosis is in the valve, the valve leaflets, or flaps, are usually stiff and stuck together, unable to move freely. When stenosis is *near* the valve, there is usually a circular growth of muscle fibers which hampers blood flow.

Some children with pulmonary stenosis have no symptoms at all; others suffer from fatigue, lightheadedness, and shortness of breath.

With or without symptoms, pulmonary stenosis can be diagnosed without difficulty. A harsh murmur is heard over the lung area and there is duplication of the second sound. The X ray may show enlargement of the heart's right ventricle, changes in the vessels in the lungs and a change in the pulmonary artery. There are usually electrocardiographic changes. The diagnosis can be confirmed by catheterization.

When stenosis is minor, no treatment is needed. In more significant narrowing, surgery is required to relieve the narrowing and prevent future damage to the heart. Childhood is the best time for the surgery.

Aortic Stenosis

The aortic valve regulates the flow of fresh, oxygen-rich blood from the left ventricle of the heart into the aorta, the great arterial trunk line of the body. Stenosis, or narrowing, of the aortic valve makes it difficult for the heart to pump blood into the aorta.

Normally the aortic valve has three cusps, or flaps. In some children, the valve has only two cusps. A bicuspid valve is more likely than a tricuspid one to become thickened and calcified, leading to significant narrowing. But obstruction to blood flow may also develop in a tricuspid valve if the cusps join together abnormally.

Most children with aortic stenosis tolerate the defect well in their early years. There may be no symptoms and general development may proceed normally. In time, however, as the valve cusps thicken, obstruction may increase and seriously interfere with heart function. Symptoms then may include fatigability and chest pain after effort.

The physician will hear a loud murmur over the aortic area. X-ray examination will show either a normal-sized heart or mild enlargement of the left ventricle—and often dilatation or enlargement of part of the aorta. There may be significant electrocardiographic changes. Catheterization can be used to confirm the diagnosis.

Surgery is done with the aid of the heart-lung machine. Sometimes, the fused portions of the valve are cut apart. In other cases, the valve is removed and replaced with a plastic substitute.

Another, less common form of aortic stenosis is subvalvular aortic stenosis, also called by the unwieldy name of idiopathic hypertrophic subaortic stenosis—the result of a membrane spread beneath the aortic valve or of a thickened muscle obstructing the blood flow out of the left ventricle.

This type of stenosis, too, may produce no symptoms early in life, but later fatigability, shortness of breath and fainting episodes may develop. The abnormality can be diagnosed by the murmur it produces and by X-ray pictures of the heart and changes in the electrocardiogram.

Drug treatment may be helpful. A compound called a beta adrenergic blocker sometimes decreases the degree of stenosis and so lightens the burden on the heart muscle. When medical treatment is inadequate, surgery may be used. Even when the operation does not result in a cure, it usually lessens the strain on the heart.

Tetralogy of Fallot

Some congenital malformations of the heart lead to the mixing of fresh and used blood, so that the blood which flows out of the heart to body tissues is oxygen-poor and bluish-red in color. This is called cyanotic heart disease ("cyanotic" comes from the Greek word for blue), and the baby is said to be a "blue baby" because of the color which develops in the fingernail beds, lips, nose tip and other areas.

Tetralogy of Fallot is the most common form of congenital

cyanotic heart disease with which a child can live for any length of time. The disease combines four different defects:

1. The pulmonary valve or the area below it is narrowed (pulmonary stenosis) and interferes with the flow of blood through the pulmonary artery to the lungs.

2. An abnormal opening in the wall between the heart's two ventricles (ventricular septal defect) allows used, unoxygenated blood in the right ventricle to mix with fresh, oxygenated blood in the left ventricle.

3. The aorta does not rise from the left ventricle but instead straddles both left and right ventricles and leaves the heart at a point just over the septal defect. Thus, the aorta receives the unhealthy mixture of oxygen-rich and oxygen-poor blood and transports it to body tissues.

4. The right ventricle is enlarged because of the extra work it must do to pump blood through the narrowed pulmonary valve.

How much the child is affected depends on the degree of obstruction to blood flow from the right ventricle to the lungs. When the obstruction is great, much of the oxygen-poor blood from the right ventricle bypasses the lungs and goes to the aorta to be distributed throughout the body. The child then may be cyanotic or blue from birth. When obstruction is relatively slight, as is often the case in early infancy, the oxygen-poor blood moves past the obstruction into the lungs, while only a small portion of it goes to the aorta; in such a case, blueness may not be seen except when the baby is crying or physically active. Occasionally, the obstruction is so mild that blueness never develops.

Except in the mildest cases, a child with Tetralogy of Fallot tends to be underdeveloped and underweight because of the inadequate oxygen supply for body tissues. Clubbing of fingers and toes (see page 20) is common. Generally, after physical exertion, a child with Tetralogy squats; this posture apparently helps him, although how or why is not known.

In diagnosing Tetralogy, the physician relies on his observation of the child's appearance, the murmur he hears through the stethoscope, X-ray examination of the heart and the results of electrocardiographic studies. Cardiac catheterization adds further confirmation and helps determine the degree of disability.

Forbidding as a combination of four defects may seem, the outlook for most children with Tetralogy today is excellent. Both medical and surgical treatment can be used.

If the heart muscle begins to fail, medication can be used to strengthen it. Often the body tries to compensate for cyanosis by increasing the number of blood cells that carry oxygen. If the increase becomes excessive, the excess cells can be removed by careful bleeding.

In most children, complete cure is possible by surgery. Usually, it is best performed in an older child or young adult; if a child is too ill to wait, a special palliative operation can give temporary relief.

The palliative operation is designed to get more blood flow to the lungs. The surgeon connects one of the arteries arising from the aorta, usually the subclavian artery, to the pulmonary artery, thereby bypassing the pulmonary valve obstruction. Then, some of the mixed oxygen-rich and oxygen-poor blood flowing through the aorta will be shunted through the pulmonary artery to the lungs for enrichment, so that more oxygen-rich blood will reach the body tissues. The operation is a safe one, and while it corrects no defects it does decrease blueness and breathing difficulties.

Later—frequently when the child is between the ages of five and twelve—a permanently corrective operation may be performed. The heart-lung machine is used. Through an incision in the right ventricle, the surgeon repairs the pulmonary valve and closes the opening in the wall between the ventricles. Results can be dramatic: a healthy pink look replaces blueness, clubbing disappears and tolerance for exercise and all physical activity increases greatly.

Transposition of the Great Vessels

This is another type of congenital cyanotic—or "blue baby"— heart disease. This is one in which the pulmonary artery is located where the aorta should be, and vice versa.

Normally, the pulmonary artery arises from the right ventricle of the heart and carries blood to the lungs for freshening. When there is transposition, the artery is attached to the left ventricle instead, and so it carries fresh blood, which has already been to the lungs, back to the lungs again.

Normally, the aorta arises from the left ventricle and carries fresh blood to body tissues. But in transposition it is attached to the right ventricle and so receives used blood and carries it to the body tissues.

Usually a child with transposition is blue at birth or within a few days afterward. Infants with transposition survive only if they are born with an additional heart defect which helps to compensate for the transposition. The additional defect may be an opening in the wall between the two ventricles (ventricular septal defect) or in the wall between the two atria (atrial septal defect). Or it may be a connection between the pulmonary artery and aorta (patent ductus arteriosus).

If one of these defects is present, there can be a mixture of fresh and used blood. The infant's survival will depend on the size of the compensating defect; in other words, on the amount of oxygenated blood the body receives.

The diagnosis of transposition is arrived at on the basis of murmurs heard, the X-ray picture and the electrocardiogram. Catheterization and angiocardiography provide confirmation.

A palliative surgical procedure may be used to help a child with transposition. An opening in the septum between the two atria is created by use of a catheter inserted into a blood vessel and maneuvered into the heart. The opening allows oxygenated blood to be rerouted to reach body tissues.

Though the procedures to date are still palliative they are often lifesaving. And there is every hope that, before long, curative techniques may be found for transposition.

Other Malformations

The eight congenital heart defects discussed above may occur in combinations. An atrial defect may be associated with a ventricular septal defect or with patent ductus arteriosus. Patent ductus arteriosus may occur in association with coarctation of the aorta or with a ventricular septal defect. And, as we saw, Tetralogy of Fallot invoives both pulmonary stenosis and ventricular septal defect.

When such combinations occur, their diagnosis usually is clear from the symptoms, physical signs and information provided by X rays, electrocardiograms and other tools. And the treatments used to correct the individual defects can be employed in combination.

In addition to the principal congenital heart defects, there are many rare ones. A few warrant brief discussion:

Truncus Arteriosus. With this defect, there is only one vessel, the aorta, to receive the blood from both ventricles of the heart. This aorta has two branches which go to the lungs.

There is yet no surgical treatment for the malformation. The outlook for an individual patient depends on how much blood is routed to the lungs by the two branches from the aorta. Some children die in infancy or early childhood; some survive into adulthood and even to middle age.

Tricuspid Atresia. This defect involves complete closure of the tricuspid valve. Blood returning from the body to the right side of the heart enters the left atrium through a large abnormal opening between the right and left atria. In the left atrium, the used blood mixes with fresh blood. The mixture goes to the left ventricle, where part is pumped into the aorta and part enters the right ventricle through an abnormal opening and goes from there to the lungs. The fraction of blood reaching the lungs is usually small, and the child is cyanotic. In some cases, an operation of the type used for Tetralogy of Fallot—connecting an artery arising from the aorta to the pulmonary artery to lead more blood to the lungs—may prove helpful.

Single Ventricle. In very rare cases, the entire ventricular septum or wall between the ventricles is missing. Thus the heart really has only a single pumping chamber. This is a most complicated malformation, and other abnormalities—such as pulmonary or aortic stenosis—almost always accompany it. Whether or not a child survives depends on the other abnormalities, since some are more compatible with life than others. Some patients with a single ventricle have been known to survive into middle age.

Ebstein's Anomaly. In this malformation, the tricuspid valve is deformed, the right ventricle is weak, and there is an atrial septal defect. A portion of blood returning from the body to the right atrium enters the left atrium through the abnormal opening. Thus, oxygen-poor and oxygen-rich blood mix and the blood pumped to the body tissues is of poor quality, producing blueness. There are various degrees of malformation. In some cases there is little chance for survival beyond infancy. Other patients live into middle age and lead almost-normal lives.

CARING FOR THE CHILD WITH A CONGENITAL HEART DEFECT

If you have a child who was born with a heart defect, you have good reason to be hopeful about his future.

During infancy, there may be no urgent need for surgery. Even a blue baby may do surprisingly well. Many babies with congenital heart defects are otherwise healthy. Your physician may well feel that it is wise, considering your child's specific problem, to wait and see how his body and circulation compensate for the defect rather than to rush into surgery.

Unless a baby is doing very poorly—gaining no weight and showing signs of a rapidly enlarging heart or other deterioration—there may be no urgent need at an early age even for such diagnostic tests as cardiac catheterization and angiocardiography.

Perhaps you are wondering whether your child is likely to develop rheumatic fever or coronary heart disease later in life because of his present heart defect. The answer is no: he will be no more susceptible than other children.

You may be worried, especially if there is cyanosis, that this will affect the brain and interfere with mental development. The reassuring fact is that the brain has priorities on the blood supply.

Nature has seen to it that the brain is nourished even if other parts of the body are not adequately supplied.

If your child has a minor defect, it is important not to treat him like an invalid. Only very rarely is it necessary to limit the activities of a child with a congenital heart defect. The child can almost always be counted on not to push beyond his capacity, not to attempt to do what he is not capable of doing. It's as if nature itself is guiding the youngster. If a child insists on engaging in some activity, in all likelihood he has the physical reserve for it.

If, in a particular case, there *is* a need to set physical limitations, your physician will spell them out. You should not try to impose additional restrictions. A child should be allowed to enjoy childhood as much as possible and to experience the psychological growth that goes with normal childhood.

It may be advisable not to let an older child with a congenital heart defect participate in highly competitive sports because he may be tempted by pride and competitiveness to overexert himself. If such a restriction is necessary, your doctor will tell you so.

A child with a congenital heart defect should, of course, receive the standard immunizations for polio, diphtheria, measles and the rest that any other child gets. If needed, dental extractions or tonsil or adenoid operations can be performed. Anesthesia can be administered safely when required.

With proper care, a child with a congenital heart defect can come safely through the various childhood diseases which afflict most youngsters.

Medical Care

As we have said, when a congenital heart defect is mild and the child does well and gives every indication of having a normal life expectancy, an operation may not be needed. He should, of course, have periodic checkups to make certain that all is going well.

Medication may or may not be required. Drugs cannot repair a defect but they can relieve symptoms or prevent complications.

And they are often valuable in keeping the condition under control until the child reaches a more suitable age for surgery.

If, for example, the heart does not contract as effectively as it should, or if an abnormal rhythm develops, medication can increase the strength of the heartbeat or convert an abnormal rhythm to a normal one. Many of the same drugs—digitalis, diuretics—often prescribed for adults with noncongenital heart problems can be given to children in adjusted dosages.

And for the child with a severe malformation that cannot now be corrected by surgery, medication offers the hope that he will reach the day when an advance in surgery will make his condition correctable.

Surgical Care

When is the best time for surgical correction of a congenital heart defect?

Generally, if a malformation does not seriously impair a child's growth and development, surgery should be delayed until he is at least beyond the age of two and preferably beyond the age of five. By then, if a defect has not repaired itself, as sometimes happens, it is not likely to do so. By then, too, the child is more fully grown, the tissues are larger and good surgical results are more likely.

In desperate circumstances, surgery is required at a very early age, even immediately after birth. While the risk of operation is greater than it would be later, it is justified because there are no real alternatives. Fortunately, such operations are often successful.

If, however, it is possible to wait until the risk is minimal, it is clearly wise to postpone surgery.

Weighing the Risk. Almost everything in life, including crossing a street, carries some risk. There is a risk in surgery for a child with a congenital defect. Once it was a high risk; it is constantly being lowered.

Today, with skilled surgeons, the chance that an operation for even a very complex defect will fail, that the child will die in the operating room or soon afterward, is less than 5 percent—less than one in twenty. And for some defects, it is less than 1 percent.

And yet this is no light decision for parents to make. How can they consider taking even a 1-in-100 or 1-in-200 chance that their child will not come through?

Before a decision is made, a number of questions concerning the specific defect must be answered. Does it threaten life immediately? If not, will it sooner or later lead to irreversible heart damage? Is there a good chance that an operation can mean a normal or near-normal life expectancy? The child's family doctor and cardiologist can help provide the answers to these and other questions so that the best possible decision can be made.

Perhaps some of our experiences with patients will help:

A murmur indicating patent ductus arteriosus was detected in a little girl when she was six. Within a week she was admitted to the hospital, and the defect was corrected. Three weeks later she was thriving, perfectly normal, free of murmur.

In another case, a two-year-old boy, blue, poorly developed, was found to have a loud heart murmur. The diagnosis was clear: severe Tetralogy of Fallot. A temporary shunting operation—attachment of the subclavian artery to the pulmonary artery to bring more blood to the lungs—was performed. Three weeks later the boy's color was healthy, he was eating well and he soon began to thrive and develop. Four years later, he had a second operation for permanent correction. He is now a healthy schoolboy, as pink as any other boy, and fully as active.

Another six-year-old boy with severe headaches and shortness of breath was found to have severely elevated blood pressure: 250/140 in the arms, lower in the legs. He had coarctation of the aorta. Six weeks after it was corrected, the blood pressure was 120/80 and he was free of symptoms.

In our practice of cardiology, 95 percent of our many young patients with congenital heart defects who have had surgery are alive and thriving today. They require frequent follow-up to make certain that all is going well, particularly those who had complex original defects, but they need little medical treatment. Generally, a child who has had a defect corrected—especially if it was not a highly complicated defect—requires no more medical treatment over the years than the average youngster.

When parents carefully weigh the reasonably small risk involved in an operation against the reasonable likelihood of a healthier and longer life for the child, the choice is usually heavily in favor of taking the small risk.

Preparing Your Child. What you tell your child about his heart condition, the necessary diagnostic tests and surgery (if that is to be done) deserves thoughtful consideration and expert advice. Your doctor will be most helpful in this area, both by talking with the child and by suggesting what you should say.

What a child imagines often is more frightening than the truth. Without going into great detail, you can tell him that his heart is not working quite as it should and that doctors now have many ways to fix it. Explain that they will examine him and probably make some tests to find out the best way to help him.

You can mention that he may have to go to a hospital so the doctors can fix his heart more easily. Assure him that he will not feel anything while they are doing this. Say that, afterward, he may hurt a bit for a short time but that he will not mind too much because he'll know that the pain will go away quickly and that he is getting better.

You can tell him that you would like him to come home right away, but that he will have to stay in the hospital for several weeks so the doctors and nurses can help him get well. Say that you know he won't mind too much because, after all, he knows he will be coming home soon and meanwhile you will come to see him regularly. Some hospitals allow parents to stay there. If you are going to do so, tell him this. Also say that he will be meeting other children in the hospital and that he will get better faster there than he could at home.

You cannot expect to erase all his fears. But by giving him an honest but not overly detailed picture, you can reduce his fears and help him face them. And the chances are very good that his morale will be higher the more gentle, loving and sympathetic you are without being despondent and tearful.

Convalescence. In most hospitals today, there is an intensive-care unit to which the patient is moved immediately after heart surgery. Here, physicians and highly trained nurses keep a twenty-four-hour watch to help assure recovery without complications, using special monitoring equipment that provides constant information about the patient's condition.

The length of time the patient must remain in the hospital after the operation depends upon the defect, its severity, the type of operation performed. On the average, the stay is about two weeks.

The length of convalescence at home is determined by the same factors. Either just before you take the child home, or during the first follow-up visit to the hospital afterward, the hospital's staff cardiologist will tell you how long convalescence is likely to take, how active you can allow the child to be while he is recuperating and what, if any, restrictions there should be in his diet.

At home, the child is again under the care of the family physician, who by then has received from the hospital team details of the hospital procedure and plans for the child's medical management.

An operation and several weeks in the hospital can be a strain on an adult, let alone on a child. Yet children are resilient. At first you may find it necessary to make adjustments in the usual household management for the sake of the child. But you may well be surprised at how soon you have to make another and happier adjustment—from treating him as a patient to treating him as a normal, healthy child.

Your doctor will guide you through the period when your child is recovering and starting back to school. There are other community resources for additional help if you need them: the hospital's social worker, the local heart-association chapter, the child's teachers, the school doctor and the school nurse.

The Child's Future. Each year thousands of children recover from successful operations for congenital heart defects, and soon begin to enjoy improved health. Many of these defects can now be cured completely. This is especially true of openings in the walls separating the heart's chambers.

Some defects can be almost, but not completely, cured. For example, pulmonary stenosis can be greatly relieved, but not completely overcome, by surgery. Even when there is only partial correction, the child usually has the prospect of a far better future, and can do much more, than before.

When correction is not complete, there may still be a murmur. But this does not mean significant impairment. Often a murmur persists even though the remaining abnormality is slight. The murmur is simply testimony to the fact that man cannot always reconstitute the structure of an imperfect heart with the same finesse with which nature produces a normal one. Still, the reconstituted heart is good.

If a defect is completely corrected, the child usually can engage in all types of normal activity after convalescence. With partial correction, he can usually be much more active than before, but some limitations may be needed—such as not engaging in competitive sports.

Understandably, parents tend to worry and to carry over some of their earlier protective attitudes. For a while after the child's operation and recovery, they may have to make a conscious effort to stop worrying excessively and being overprotective. It is well worth the effort, for the child needs new opportunities now to develop mind and body.

No two cases are exactly alike. What each child can do and should be encouraged to do after heart surgery is best determined by the child's own doctor. The doctor will have valuable advice, too, about vocational planning so that the child can be guided toward a career that will not make excessive physical demands on him.

But the most important thing to remember is that the outlook for his future is good.

CONGENITAL DEFECTS IN ADULTS

Effective treatment is available today for many adults—middle-aged as well as young adults—with congenital heart defects.

Some heart defects produce no symptoms early in life but may do so later. Sometimes, in the past, defects went undetected during the early years for lack of symptoms. In some cases, defects were diagnosed at an early age but effective surgery was not then available.

If an adult has a defect that produces few, relatively mild symptoms which can be controlled with medication, and if there is no indication that irreversible heart damage may be occurring, surgery may not be needed.

But now, if there is need for operation—if the problem is becoming increasingly severe—the very same surgical approaches used for children can be and are being applied effectively to adults.

[4]

Rheumatic Fever:
The Disease That
"Bites" the Heart

One of man's most common "minor" ailments is the sore throat. There are many different disease organisms that can infect the throat and make it sore. When the infection is caused by one particular organism, called Group A hemolytic streptococcus, there is a special risk.

In about 3 percent of cases, particularly among children, a strep sore throat is followed, after an interval of several weeks, by an attack of a different kind called rheumatic fever.

Rheumatic fever is so named because it produces pain and inflammation in joints such as the knees, wrists or elbows. Often, especially in the young, joint symptoms may be so mild and brief as to pass unnoticed or be labeled "growing pains."

The most serious aspect of rheumatic fever is not its effects on the joints, but its ability to produce an inflammation of the heart which may leave one or more of the heart valves damaged. This damage is rarely serious after a first attack of rheumatic fever, but the person who suffers one attack often becomes susceptible to repeated attacks, which may lead to further damage.

Rheumatic heart disease has been the most common heart

disease of childhood and youth. Currently, it affects more than one million people in the United States. Fortunately, many children and adults with rheumatic heart disease can lead normal lives; many others now are being helped by new medical and surgical treatments. Happily, too, there has been great progress in recent years in preventing rheumatic heart disease through prevention of rheumatic fever.

WHO GETS RHEUMATIC FEVER?

The great majority of first attacks of rheumatic fever occur in children between the ages of five and fifteen. Such attacks are seldom seen below the age of three and are rare in adults.

Rheumatic fever is most common in temperate climates. It is relatively rare in tropical and frigid areas, though why is not clear.

The incidence of the disease reaches a peak in late winter and early spring, much as does the incidence of strep infections.

Socio-economic factors have long been indicted. Poor housing, crowding, dampness and poor diet seem to be predisposing factors. Rheumatic fever also is more likely to occur in families with a previous history of the disease—perhaps because of some hereditary susceptibility, but more likely because of the environment, diet and other social and economic conditions shared by members of these families. If one child has had rheumatic fever, there is about a one-in-ten chance that another child in the family may develop it unless special precautions are taken.

Fortunately, rheumatic fever today seems to be milder than it once was. Only thirty years or so ago, there were entire small hospitals given over to the care of young children with rheumatic fever. Now, it is unusual to see more than a few such patients even in a large hospital.

THE NATURE OF RHEUMATIC FEVER

Rheumatic fever, as we have said, is triggered by a strep infection—but not immediately. The patient has a sore throat and fever for several days, recovers, feels well for one or two weeks, then suddenly develops rheumatic fever.

It is believed that the strep germ itself does *not* cause the rheumatic fever; it does not directly invade the joints. Instead, as the germ multiplies in the nose and throat, products are formed which are absorbed into the body. Some people have a reaction to these products similar to an allergy. And it is this allergic reaction which causes the inflammation of the joints. The interval between the sore throat and the onset of rheumatic fever is the length of time it takes the body to develop the allergic reaction.

Rheumatic fever may produce painful, hot swelling in one or several joints; the knees, wrists and elbows are those most often involved. The attack may start in one or two joints, and then an additional joint may become inflamed every few days. As the new joints are affected, those that were first inflamed start to improve. For all of these joints, the pains will, in time, disappear.

In younger children, especially those under ten, rheumatic fever symptoms may be deceptively mild. Instead of red, swollen painful joints, there may be only vague aching in the arms and legs. In some cases there may be low-grade fever, failure to gain weight, repeated nosebleeds.

Sometimes the sole indication of rheumatic fever is Saint Vitus's dance. The first sign of Saint Vitus's dance is often clumsiness; the child may spill food and drop things. When Saint Vitus's dance becomes more severe, the child may be unable to control muscles of the face, tongue, arms or legs, and may twist and jerk. But this affliction is only temporary for rheumatic-fever victims.

THE HEART COMPLICATION

It has been said of rheumatic fever that it "licks the joints but bites the heart."

Since the joint pains, involuntary movements and other symptoms almost invariably disappear, rheumatic fever might be considered an uncomfortable but not particularly important disease —except for one thing: rheumatic fever can also inflame one or more of the valves in the heart. These valves are designed to open, let blood through, and then close to prevent backflow. Inflammation from rheumatic fever can distort a valve. Though healing follows the inflammation, the scar tissue that forms may interfere with valve function.

Rheumatic fever causes two kinds of valve deformities. With one, the valve leaflets become separated so that complete closure is no longer possible and leakage occurs. With the other, the leaflets become fused, or joined, so that the valve no longer opens completely and blood flow through it is impaired. Sometimes, a single valve may show some of each type of deformity.

The severity of symptoms of rheumatic fever is no guide to the extent of damage that may be inflicted on a heart valve. Mild rheumatic fever may leave considerable damage. On the other hand, an episode of rheumatic fever may involve severe arthritis or severe Saint Vitus's dance and yet be followed by complete recovery without evidence of a heart problem.

After an initial attack of rheumatic fever, 10 to 20 percent of children have some heart-valve damage, but often it is minor. The outlook for them—and for those who escape heart damage completely—is excellent if repeated attacks are prevented, and they can be. We will discuss this preventive treatment later, but first let us consider what can be done to treat a case of rheumatic fever.

TREATING RHEUMATIC FEVER

There is no magic drug to cure rheumatic fever, but there are measures that help speed the patient toward recovery.

Once rheumatic fever is present, the rheumatic activity is not likely to be affected by antibacterial medication. But many patients at this point still harbor streptococci in their throats or deep inside tonsil or adenoid tissue. To eradicate these organisms, antibiotic treatment is begun at once. Penicillin may be given by mouth four times a day for a ten-day period, or a single injection of long-acting penicillin may be used.

Since reduction of activity helps to relieve inflammatory conditions, patients with rheumatic fever are put to bed, sometimes in a hospital, sometimes at home. At one time, bed rest for many months was common. But with the more effective measures available today, prolonged bed rest and severe restriction of physical activity are unnecessary and even undesirable.

For a rheumatic-fever child with no heart involvement, bed rest is usually continued only until the doctor finds, by means of a simple test, that the blood-sedimentation rate has become normal. This test measures the time required for blood cells in a standard amount of blood to settle. If the rate has returned to normal, it's a signal that the disease is under control.

If a child has indications of heart involvement—such as rapid pulse and enlargement of the heart—bed rest is usually continued for three to four weeks, until these indications as well as the sedimentation rate have become normal.

During the bed-rest period, the child may be allowed to use the bathroom and sit at the table for meals. As he improves, quiet play about the house may also be allowed.

Aspirin is valuable. In addition to lowering fever, it helps to relieve acute inflammatory symptoms of the joints and to return the sedimentation rate to normal. But very large amounts of aspirin are no more effective than moderate amounts, so do not be tempted to give your child more than the doctor prescribes.

When the heart is involved, hormones such as cortisone or ACTH (pituitary hormone) may be prescribed. Some doctors feel that these agents help to put a lid on inflammatory processes and so may minimize complications. Hormone treatment may lead to side effects such as puffy face, weight gain, excess hair and acne when continued for long periods, but these undesirable effects disappear once medication is stopped.

When a child must remain in bed for several weeks, diet should be palatable and nutritious but the child should not be overfed. Excessive caloric intake and weight gain are to be avoided. There should be adequate lighting for reading in bed. If at all possible, the child should follow a modified course of study prescribed by his regular teacher, or by a special home or hospital teacher, so that he does not become disturbed about falling behind his classmates.

During this time we urge the parents of our patients to tender as much love and emotional support as they possibly can. No child likes to be confined indoors and not be allowed to participate in normal activities. The situation is a trying one, and a youngster at this time, more than ever, needs parental reassurance.

As recovery proceeds, there should be a gradual, rather than a sudden, return to activity to minimize muscle aches and fatigue.

LET YOUR CHILD BE NORMAL

Almost all recovered rheumatic-fever patients can lead normal or near-normal lives. Yet many children who have had an attack are pushed into fear-ridden, sedentary lives by well-meaning but misinformed parents.

Although, thanks to continuous prophylactic treatment, recurrences of the disease are now rare, it is often difficult to convince anxious patients that this is so.

There are still too many children like the boy who, after a single rheumatic-fever incident which did not affect his heart, was nevertheless considered an invalid by his mother. He was never permitted to go out on the playground. He ate his lunch in a classroom. His mother requested that he be excused from extra-curricular activities at school. She would not permit him to have a bicycle or skates. Finally, a concerned school nurse took the boy to a crippled-children's clinic. Clinic physicians had to reassure the boy and his mother for five years before he could begin to lead the life of the normally healthy youngster he was.

Recently Dr. John H. Kennell and a team of investigators at Case Western Reserve University, Cleveland, made a two-year study of sixty-three young rheumatic fever patients and their parents. The study concluded that the parents continue to treat these children with kid gloves, as if recurrences of rheumatic fever could be caused by cold weather or exercise, instead of only streptococcal infections.

More than two-thirds of the mothers of young patients with normal hearts reported to the investigators that they imposed on their children restrictions that might have been thought necessary before antibiotics: no running, bike-riding, rough sports or games. The children were also overdressed in winter.

The parents of adolescents were found to be worrying unnecessarily about what would happen to the youngsters when they reached adulthood. They were determined to find sedentary occupations for them. Some parents doubted their children's suitability for marriage. And many parents of girls worried about the strains of pregnancy and childbirth.

The problem seems to be that rheumatic fever is still equated with heart disease and death. It is true that, prior to the early 1950's, it was a crippler and killer, a major cause of hospital admissions and of death. But it is not now.

Unless your child's heart has been very seriously damaged—and your physician will tell you if it is—he is likely to be able to live a normal life and will do best if permitted to.

PREVENTING RECURRENCES

A child who has had a bout of rheumatic fever must not be allowed to have additional strep infections. After an initial attack of rheumatic fever, susceptibility to the disease is increased. We know now that the younger a child is when a first attack of rheumatic fever occurs, the more likely recurrences are unless precautions are taken: without precautions, recurrences develop in as many as 90 percent of patients who have had an initial attack before the age of ten. Furthermore, if the heart was not affected in the first attack, it may be in subsequent attacks, and if there was damage in the initial attack, repeated episodes may add to it. But the longer a child is well after an attack, the better his chance of avoiding a recurrence.

For these reasons, continuous prophylactic or preventive treatment against strep infections is vitally important. Antibacterial treatment—oral penicillin, long-acting penicillin by injection, or sulfa drugs—may be used. All are effective. At present, oral penicillin twice a day is the most widely used.

There is no question about the value of such prophylactic

treatment. Studies have demonstrated that where once, about twenty years ago, 50 to 75 percent of rheumatic fever patients had recurrences, now, with regular prophylaxis, the recurrence is down to 3 percent and may well go lower.

Is it necessary to continue prophylaxis year-round? It is. While strep infections are more common in winter and spring months, they can occur at any season.

How long must prophylaxis be maintained? The risk of acquiring a strep infection is present throughout life. Rheumatic fever itself tends to be more recurrent during youth; attacks are less frequent after the age of thirty. But the safest procedure is to continue prophylaxis indefinitely, especially if there has been some damage to the heart. Some physicians may make exceptions in adult patients, particularly in those who have no heart problem and who have had no rheumatic-fever recurrences for many years.

PREVENTING THE FIRST RHEUMATIC FEVER ATTACK

Strep infections are common but can be treated effectively. If the strep germs are destroyed by antibiotic treatment before allergic reaction develops, there is little likelihood that rheumatic fever will follow. In fact, there is evidence that rheumatic fever may be prevented even when antibiotic treatment is started as late as the ninth day after the onset of a strep infection.

The problem is how to recognize a strep throat. Not every sore throat is a strep throat. The chances are that a child does *not* have a strep infection if his only complaint is hoarseness or a cough. A child can have a strep infection without having a sore throat—and that somewhat complicates the problem.

The American Heart Association recommends certain procedures for you to follow to make sure you are doing all you can to protect your child from rheumatic fever.

If your child gets a sore throat and has any of the indications suggested in the following seven questions, phone your doctor at once and be ready to give him the answers to all the questions.

1. Did the sore throat come on suddenly?

2. Does your youngster complain that his throat hurts most when he swallows?

3. Does it hurt him under the angle of his jaw when you press gently with your fingers? Are the glands in his neck swollen?

4. Does he have a fever? How much? (Usually a strep infection brings a fever of 101 to 104.)

5. Does your child complain of headache?

6. Is he nauseated? Has he vomited?

7. Has he been in contact with anyone who has had a sore throat or scarlet fever? (Any child who has been exposed to scarlet fever should see his doctor for preventive treatment even if he does not have a sore throat.)

The answers to these questions can help your doctor decide if he should examine your child for a possible strep infection.

RHEUMATIC HEART DISEASE

During an acute rheumatic-fever attack, the physician may hear a heart murmur.

As we have said, not all murmurs indicate a heart problem. Some are innocent and may have been present but undetected before the rheumatic-fever incident. Some murmurs that occur during the acute stage of rheumatic fever are simply the result of fever and anemia and disappear when these symptoms depart. Still other murmurs indicate that the heart valves are stretched and swollen, and they will stop when the valves return to normal within a few weeks or months.

After a rheumatic-fever episode is over, the physician examines the patient periodically to determine if a murmur heard during the episode has disappeared. If it persists, he considers whether it is a normal murmur or one that indicates rheumatic heart disease. If it does indicate heart disease, he has other questions to answer: Has there been mild, moderate or severe injury to a heart valve? Which valve, or valves, are involved?

The most frequently involved valve is the mitral, but the problem may lie with the aortic valve. Sometimes, both mitral and aortic valves are affected.

When the Mitral Valve Is Affected

The mitral valve controls the movement of blood from the left atrium, where the blood arrives freshened from the lungs, to the left ventricle, which pumps the blood out into the aorta.

During an acute rheumatic-fever attack, areas of the mitral valve may thicken so that the valve cannot close properly. Sometimes when the attack subsides, the valve returns to normal size and regains its ability to close, but in other cases there is permanent impairment.

When the valve cannot close properly, there is backward leakage, or regurgitation, of blood, from the ventricle to the atrium. The valve deformity may be mild and the regurgitation small, so that the patient will experience no difficulty at all during a normal lifetime.

But with severe regurgitation, fatigue and weakness develop. The physician can hear a loud, high-pitched murmur. He can also detect, through X-ray pictures and electrocardiographic patterns, enlargement of the left ventricle: the ventricle enlarges to try to push more blood out to the body to compensate for that which is regurgitated. Faulty closure of the mitral valve is called mitral insufficiency.

The most common potentially troublesome mitral-valve defect is stenosis, inability to *open* properly. With stenosis, the flow of blood from the atrium into the ventricle is reduced. Since the atrium, in contracting, cannot push most of its blood through to the ventricle, blood pressure is built up in the chamber and the pressure rises. The pressure is transmitted back through the pulmonary veins to the lungs, and lung functioning is affected.

At first there may be labored breathing only on severe exertion, but gradually the ability to exercise becomes more limited. There may be spitting of blood as small blood vessels in the lungs and airways rupture, having become engorged with blood from the back pressure. In mitral stenosis, too, the right ventricle enlarges as the pressure to the lungs is transmitted back from them to the heart chamber.

The physician, through his stethoscope, can hear characteristic sounds of mitral stenosis. There are typical abnormalities of size and shape to be seen on X-rays. Electrocardiographic findings also are helpful in diagnosis.

When the Aortic Valve Is Involved

The aortic valve controls the flow of blood from the left ventricle into the great artery, the aorta. It, too, may be affected by rheumatic fever, so that it fails either to open or to close normally.

With incomplete closure, there is an added burden on the left ventricle. Because blood leaks backward through the valve, the ventricle must pump harder to maintain adequate circulation throughout the body, and thus it enlarges. The patient usually experiences no symptoms from incomplete closure, or aortic insufficiency, until the ventricle, after many years of the added burden of work, begins to lose its ability to pump effectively. Then heart failure develops and leads to such symptoms as labored breathing and fluid accumulation (see Chapter 7).

Aortic insufficiency can be diagnosed by the physician even if the patient has no overt symptoms. There is a telltale heart murmur, and there are additional clues in the size of the heart, the quality of the pulse and the level of blood pressure.

In aortic stenosis, the leaflets of the valve become fused and cannot open properly. If the size of the valve opening is significantly reduced, there is a greater build-up of pressure within the left ventricle to force the blood through, and as a result the left ventricle thickens. Because of the added work, the heart muscle needs more oxygen, which must be supplied by the coronary arteries which branch off the aorta. But with all the hard work of the ventricle, the blood flow into the aorta may be less than normal—and so, therefore, will be the flow through the coronary arteries

Symptoms of aortic stenosis are related to the decreased flow of blood through the coronary arteries and through other arteries which branch off from the aorta and lead to the brain. The most important symptoms are chest pain and fainting. The chest pain is like that of angina pectoris (see Chapter 9), and is brought on by physical exertion and relieved by rest. Fainting, or lightheadedness, associated with reduced blood flow to the brain, occurs particularly after exertion.

Treatment for Rheumatic Heart Disease

Valve deformities resulting from rheumatic fever vary greatly in degree. A valve opening can be reduced to as little as *one-half* its original size without significant consequences. When the reduction is greater, a murmur is apparent, but even then it may be not until the valve opening is reduced to *one-fourth* its original size that the work load on the heart is materially increased.

Similarly, slight regurgitation through a valve that does not close completely is usually of little importance. There must be a large amount of regurgitation before the burden on the heart becomes significantly greater.

Thus, many patients with mild rheumatic heart disease sail through normal lifetimes without any difficulties at all. And some with moderate disease experience only minor, nondisabling symptoms.

On the other hand, severe disease may cause disability early in life.

And sometimes disability may develop abruptly. For example, a woman had had several attacks of rheumatic fever in childhood which left her with mitral stenosis that caused no difficulty. She had a definite murmur, but she was able to lead a normal life and went through three pregnancies with only minor problems. Then, in her late thirties, she went into heart failure quite suddenly. The failure was overcome by medical treatment, but she remained moderately disabled. At that point surgery was used to overcome the stenosis, and she has been free of trouble since.

Medical Treatment. Medical treatment for rheumatic heart

disease is directed against complications. For heart failure—loss of the heart's pumping efficiency—the basic elements of treatment are digitalis to strengthen the heart and diuretics and salt restriction to promote elimination of excess fluids (see Chapter 7).

An irregular heart rhythm may develop with mitral stenosis. It is called atrial fibrillation. Instead of contracting, the atria, the upper chambers of the heart, twitch. Although this may sound ominous, blood still flows from the upper chambers to the ventricles. Atrial fibrillation is thus not a lethal complication, but it does reduce the working efficiency of the heart. The fibrillation can be converted to normal rhythmic contraction with medication such as quinidine.

Surgical Treatment. In 1949, a surgical technique for successfully correcting mitral stenosis was reported. Since then, operations have been developed for correcting other valve deformities.

In determining whether surgery is advisable, the physician considers the patient's symptoms and response to medical treatment. He also bears in mind the difficulties and risks of operation.

When a mitral or aortic valve is obstructed, it is relatively easy for a surgeon to correct the deformity. With the aid of the heart-lung machine, he can open the heart and inspect the valve. He can then snip apart the fused leaflets of the valve to allow better blood flow.

When mitral- or aortic-valve leakage is the problem, the surgeon replaces the valve with an artificial valve consisting of a small disk that moves in a little cage. The operation, also performed with the aid of a heart-lung machine, takes about three hours. Afterward the patient is carefully monitored. Usually he is eating and drinking well within seventy-two hours and can go home within two weeks.

The operation to replace a valve is somewhat riskier than surgery to repair a stenosed valve, and so there is usually more caution about using it. However, when the operation is needed the risk is well justified, for it can be profoundly beneficial, preventing invalidism and even saving life.

We would like to emphasize that surgery is not by any means an inevitable requirement for patients with rheumatic heart disease. In our practice of cardiology, we have followed many patients with mitral- and aortic-valve deformities for long periods—twenty years and more—and they have done well without surgery. They have had no worsening of signs and symptoms, nor, it seems, are they ever likely to.

On the other hand, for some patients, modern surgery—and it is constantly improving—is of great value. We have been following for periods up to fifteen years more than 1,200 patients who benefited greatly from surgery. More than 600 underwent operations to correct mitral stenosis, about 300 had mitral-valve replacement, and about 300 had aortic-valve replacement.

In the past, prosthetic—artificial—valves sometimes caused problems. Earlier valves were not so effective as those now used. The materials used sometimes led to formation of blood clots which could break loose and travel to a coronary, brain, or leg artery and cause trouble. Happily, such clot formation now is rare. Another complication, anemia, sometimes occurred as a result of mechanical destruction of red blood cells by artificial valves. This complication, too, is becoming rare.

Thus, there has been much progress in the treatment of rheumatic disease. Surgical correction of valve deformities is a significant advance; medical treatment of rheumatic fever has even wider usefulness; and the prevention of rheumatic fever is more basic still.

Some Questions and Answers

A patient with rheumatic heart disease has many specific questions he would like answered. These are among the most common:

Can I keep on working? Very probably. In fact, most people with heart disease can and should do some kind of work. The kind of work you can do will, of course, depend on your individual condition, and your physician can advise you specifically about this.

Can I get help in finding a suitable job? If your doctor has recommended that you change your job for a more suitable one, he may be able to direct you to services that will be helpful. Some local heart associations maintain work-classification units staffed by professional personnel who study individual patients and suggest work best suited to them. Every state has an office of the Division of Vocational Rehabilitation which provides guidance and training for people with limited physical capacities; your doctor or the local heart association can help you get in touch with that office.

Should I move to another climate to avoid getting rheumatic fever again? That is not necessary. The need is to prevent strep infections which cause rheumatic fever, and you can do this by taking the medication prescribed by your doctor.

Is it safe for a woman with rheumatic heart disease to have children? Usually, yes, if she follows her physician's instructions. If there *is* any possibility of undue risk for her in undertaking pregnancy and in caring for a family, the doctor can tell her that, too. (For a discussion of pregnancy and heart disease, see Chapter 8.)

Will my children inherit rheumatic fever from me? While there may be some inherited proneness to rheumatic fever, the disease does *not* occur unless there has been a strep infection. To be safe, make certain that any member of your family with a sore throat or other symptoms that may indicate a strep infection is seen promptly by your doctor. Refer back to page 57 for guidance on this.

Do I need a special diet for rheumatic heart disease? Probably not—unless you are overweight or your salt intake should be limited. Extra weight makes extra work for any heart and is detrimental when there is a heart problem. If you need to lose weight, avoid your neighbor's diet or diets you see in newspapers and magazines. Let your doctor advise you about a diet suitable for you. If your salt intake needs to be limited, your doctor will advise you about the extent of limitation and how best to achieve it.

Can I have dental work done? Yes, with simple precautions. Tooth extractions and some other dental procedures may cause bacteria to get loose, enter the blood stream and be carried to the heart. Such bacteria usually are harmless to normal hearts but sometimes may infect and inflame a heart which has been affected by rheumatic fever. Your doctor and dentist can consult so that suitable precautions can be taken. If you are using penicillin regularly to prevent rheumatic fever, you will require larger doses at the time of dental work.

Is there any possibility that a vaccine may be developed to prevent strep infections? Yes. Several groups of researchers are working on the problem. The key seems to lie in a material called the M protein, found in the cell walls of strep bacteria. When an infectious organism invades the body and multiplies, the body responds by producing substances called antibodies which attack and eventually may overcome the organisms. Injection of the M protein beforehand appears to excite the body to produce antibodies which would then be immediately available to combat invading strep and perhaps prevent infection. Each type of strep has its own M protein. There are fifty-odd types of Group A strep. But less than ten of these are responsible for more than two-thirds of strep infections, and so some researchers believe that a vaccine made up of perhaps six to eight M proteins could lead to a marked drop in the number of strep infections.

[5]

Heart Infections

Like any other organ of the body, the heart may be directly invaded by disease organisms. Among these organisms are the spirochetes which produce syphilis; staphylococcal, streptococcal and other bacteria; and viruses including those causing influenza, mumps and measles.

CARDIOVASCULAR SYPHILIS

Cardiovascular syphilis is a peculiar disease, both in the way it develops and in the long time it takes to manifest itself. Today it is both curable and preventable. Education, public health measures, early diagnosis and modern treatment have led to a sharp decrease in the incidence of cardiovascular syphilis, but it is still a disease to be reckoned with.

It is a complication of syphilis—and syphilis itself is peculiar. Arising as the result of sexual contact with an infected person, syphilis first manifests itself in the form of a sore, usually on the genitals, three to six weeks after contact. The sore disappears even

66

without treatment. But then, in another three to six weeks, syphilis manifests itself again with a rash which may appear anywhere on the body and may be accompanied by fever or sore throat, or both. And again, even without treatment, these symptoms disappear.

At any time up to this point, and even later, treatment with antibiotics can eradicate syphilis. But if there is no treatment, the disease remains even as the symptoms vanish. It goes underground for many years. Subtly, progressively, it attacks various organs, such as the liver, brain and spinal cord. And it may attack the cardiovascular system.

The spirochetes which enter the blood stream have a tendency, for unknown reasons, to concentrate in the first portion of the aorta, the great trunk artery. The area becomes chronically inflamed.

Usually, ten to twenty years go by after the original syphilis infection before cardiovascular syphilis becomes evident. Because of this long period of development, syphilitic heart disease is most frequent in adults between the ages of thirty-five and fifty-five, although it has been known to develop in people as young as twenty and as old as seventy. It is much more common in men than in women.

As a result of chronic inflammation, the aorta widens. The widening itself usually produces no symptoms. But as the widening progresses, the wall of the aorta may become thinned out at some point, and an aneurysm—a ballooned-out area similar to the bubble that sometimes appears on an automobile tire wall—may develop.

Sometimes an aneurysm produces no symptoms. But if it presses on nearby structures, the patient may cough and experience chest pain and breathing difficulty. And the danger is that it may burst, leading to sudden death.

In about one-quarter of the patients with cardiovascular syphilis, the aortic valve also is affected. The valve does not close completely, and some blood leaks back from the aorta into the heart. This adds to the pumping burden of the left ventricle, which thickens and enlarges to meet the challenge. In time, under the extra load, the ventricle may lose its pumping efficiency, and congestive heart failure then follows.

In some cases, the coronary arteries may be affected, too, at the points where they branch off from the aorta. They may become narrowed by inflammation, thus reducing the amount of blood flowing to the heart muscle and producing angina pectoris, the chest pain associated with inadequate nutrition of the heart muscle.

It has been well-established that early and adequate treatment for syphilis, usually with penicillin, greatly reduces the likelihood of heart complications. There is now evidence that penicillin treatment directed at the syphilis may prolong the life of a patient who already has an inflamed aorta, aortic-valve deformity and coronary-artery involvement.

It was once thought that when cardiovascular syphilis had reached the point of producing congestive heart failure, the outlook was poor. Now, however, with use of medications employed for congestive heart failure from any cause (see Chapter 7), survival for ten years and more is not unusual.

Angina pectoris caused by cardiovascular syphilis is a serious problem, but long survivals have been reported. The chest pain usually responds to nitroglycerin, the medication that is commonly used for angina pectoris from other causes (see page 110).

Many aneurysms can now be treated successfully by surgery, thanks to the development of artificial vessels that can be grafted on to replace a weakened, ballooning area of aorta. Today, too, an aortic valve hopelessly diseased by cardiovascular syphilis can be replaced with an artificial valve.

BACTERIAL ENDOCARDITIS

Endocarditis is a heart-valve infection. The infection may spread to the heart from a starting site elsewhere in the body or may begin within the heart.

Under certain conditions, infection may begin in the heart as the result of invasion by bacteria which ordinarily are relatively innocuous. Usually, this happens when there has been previous damage to a heart valve, such as in rheumatic heart disease or congenital heart disease. The most common infecting agent is the green streptococcus (*Streptococcus viridans*). Green strep appears to be an innocent occupant of the mouth, and though it may occasionally get into the blood stream, it is usually readily eliminated by body defenses. But when it finds a weak area, such as a damaged valve, green strep can lodge there, multiply and form "vegetations" on the valve. The vegetations consist of bacteria, trapped blood cells and other material.

The patient experiences fever which may reach a daily peak of almost 104, chills, loss of appetite, and weakness. Anemia may develop and intensify weakness and fatigability. Crops of tiny red spots may appear on the skin and mucous membranes. New murmurs may develop or previously existing ones may change in character as a valve is slowly destroyed by the vegetation. The vegetation also makes it easier for small blood clots to form; these may tear loose, reach distant arteries and cause damage to brain, legs or abdominal organs.

Until 1943, bacterial endocarditis was 99 percent fatal. Then the newly discovered drug penicillin proved capable of curing many cases of endocarditis due to green strep. And with the availability of other antibiotics, endocarditis now has become 90 percent curable.

Treatment aims at total elimination of infection just as quickly as possible to prevent damage to valves and development of clots. Treatment is intensive—usually carried out in a hospital. Generally, medication is given by injection into a vein. Sometimes, in order to destroy the bacteria, as many as 50 million units of penicillin daily (as against the usual 1 million units per day), along with streptomycin and other antibiotics, may be needed. And treatment may be continued for as long as six weeks to make certain that organisms deeply embedded in valve vegetations are destroyed.

The best way to deal with endocarditis, of course, is to prevent it. Since people with congenital heart disease or rheumatic heart disease are in danger of developing endocarditis, they should be protected whenever they are exposed to the possibility of bacteria circulating in the blood stream. With large doses of penicillin or other antibiotics, they can be protected during dental extractions, tonsillectomy and other procedures in the nose and throat area. They can be protected similarly during childbirth and during surgical and other procedures elsewhere in the body.

In the past, some patients cured of the disease have died a few years after treatment because of progressive valve deformity. It is now possible to save some of these patients by replacement of the diseased valve with an artificial device.

ACUTE PERICARDITIS

Acute pericarditis is an inflammation of the pericardial sac which encloses the heart.

Infectious agents, including viruses and various bacteria, can invade the sac and produce the inflammation. Pericarditis may also develop as a complication when the heart itself is inflamed because of rheumatic fever or heart attack. It may be the result, too, of direct injury, as from a stab or gunshot wound.

The most common infectious agent is a virus. Typically, the patient has had a cold or other respiratory infection. Then, on top of the fever and general malaise, comes chest pain. The pain is aggravated by breathing, coughing and lying down. It may shoot out to the back, shoulder, abdomen. Sometimes it seems much like that of angina pectoris, suggesting coronary heart disease. Acute pericarditis can be a frightening experience.

The physician is able to diagnose the condition readily by the rubbing sound he can hear through his stethoscope. It is a friction rub, indicating that the layers of the pericardial sac are rubbing against each other. There are also characteristic changes on the electrocardiogram.

There is no effective agent to knock out the viruses causing the trouble, but the body's defenses will do that in time. Meanwhile, bed rest helps. The patient can be made comfortable with pain-relievers. In severe cases, steroids—cortisonelike drugs—may be used. The illness may last from one to three weeks, and the patient usually recovers completely.

Acute pericarditis caused by bacterial rather than viral infection has become much less common since the advent of antibiotics. It does, however, still occur, and most often the organisms are staph, strep, or pneumococci. The symptoms are high fever, chest pain and friction rub. For bacterial pericarditis, antibiotics can be used to help speed recovery.

A tuberculous form of acute pericarditis may occur when tuberculosis is present elsewhere in the body, usually in the lungs or nearby lymph nodes. Usually in this case there is no chest pain but the patient experiences weight loss, fever, night sweats and loss of appetite. Tuberculous pericarditis is treated with anti-TB drugs such as isoniazid and para-aminosalicylic acid, and the chances for recovery are excellent.

Commonly, acute pericarditis occurs in the "dry" form we have been discussing. But sometimes it is accompanied by effusion: fluid accumulates between the layers of the pericardial sac. The heart then appears enlarged on X-ray film. There are changes in heart sounds and in the pulse and the electrocardiogram.

If a great amount of fluid accumulates, it may compress the heart enough so that the flow of blood returning from the body to the heart is impeded. This is called cardiac tamponade.

When cardiac tamponade is severe, the removal of even a small amount of fluid brings quick relief. A needle is inserted through the chest wall into the pericardial sac to withdraw the fluid. The procedure, called pericardiocentesis, is not nearly as formidable as it sounds. It is usually carried out by a heart surgeon, who follows the changes which appear on the patient's electrocardiogram as he slowly advances the needle. The changes tell him when he has reached exactly the right area for fluid withdrawal.

Although acute pericarditis is painful, most patients recover without any permanent aftereffects.

CHRONIC CONSTRICTIVE PERICARDITIS

The pericardial sac eases the action of the heart by providing fluid that acts as a kind of lubricant. It also confines the heart and thus prevents too sudden dilation.

But if the pericardial sac becomes abnormally thickened and

loses its flexibility, it can act like a rigid container around the heart, seriously interfering with the heart's work. This is what happens in chronic constrictive pericarditis.

Often the reason for it is unknown. Sometimes tuberculosis is a cause. Occasionally bacterial and viral pericarditis may produce it. Rheumatic fever rarely, if ever, is responsible.

Chronic constrictive pericarditis is three times as common in men as in women and occurs most often between the second and fifth decades of life.

Its major effect is to interfere with the normal relaxation and expansion of the heart between beats. As a result, the return of blood from the body through the vein system to the heart is impeded. Pressure builds up in the veins and, characteristically, veins in the neck become distended. Fluid accumulates in the legs and in the abdominal cavity. The liver enlarges. Loss of weight, loss of appetite, and weakness are common complaints.

Sometimes constrictive pericarditis is readily diagnosable. Calcium deposits in the sac may show up on X-ray film. Clues may be obtained, too, from heart size and rate and from heart sounds. Sometimes, however, distinguishing pericarditis from right-sided heart failure resulting from valve disease and from other conditions may require special diagnostic studies such as heart catheterization and angiocardiography (see page 24 for both).

The treatment for constrictive pericarditis is surgical. The very first operations on the human heart were *emergency* procedures for stab wounds. The surgical treatment of constrictive pericarditis was the first *elective* procedure and stands as a milestone in modern heart surgery.

Before the operation, the patient is relieved of large fluid accumulations by means of diuretic drugs and, if necessary, by pericardiocentesis. If tuberculosis has been found, the patient is treated with antituberculosis drugs for at least ten days prior to surgery.

In the operation, called pericardiectomy, the entire constricting sac is removed. Afterward, the patient is vastly improved. Abdominal and ankle fluid accumulations disappear; the liver returns to normal; exercise tolerance becomes normal. We have seen patients who were dying return to vigorous jobs after surgery.

ACUTE MYOCARDITIS

Myocarditis is an inflammation of the heart muscle. It may occur as a complication of rheumatic fever or of bacterial, viral and other infections elsewhere in the body. Once it was a dreaded complication of diphtheria, but immunization has made diphtheria rare now. Still, common communicable diseases of childhood, particularly mumps, are occasionally followed by myocarditis. The heart-muscle inflammation may also be triggered by influenza, viral hepatitis, infectious mononucleosis and acute bacterial endocarditis. It may also occur as the result of drug reactions, poisoning and heat stroke.

In myocarditis, the heart becomes enlarged and the heart muscle flabby. Chest discomfort, labored breathing, palpitations and racing pulse are common. The physician is aided in diagnosis by these indications and also by changes in heart sounds, the enlargement of the heart shown on X-ray films and electrocardiographic changes.

Strict bed rest is required during the active stage of the disease. If the myocarditis stems from bacterial infection, antibacterial drugs are used to eliminate the infection. The patient is made as comfortable as possible. Fever is reduced with aspirin and tepid sponge baths. Dietary and fluid intakes are adjusted. Sedatives may be used to help control restlessness. Other medications may be employed to provide symptom relief.

In a rare case, there may be sudden death from heart failure. But most patients recover—and the great majority of those who recover regain normal function of the heart.

[6]

High Blood Pressure
and Heart Disease

High blood pressure, also called hypertension, is a common problem. It afflicts an estimated 17 million Americans between the ages of eighteen and seventy-nine, roughly one of every six adults.

If you know that you have hypertension, it is probably because your physician has told you so. Rarely does a person suspect it from symptoms For hypertension is a stealthy disease. It seldom produces any distinctive symptoms, although there is a common misconception that it does.

The important thing about hypertension is the damage it can do to the heart, the arteries, the kidneys and the brain if it is uncontrolled over long periods.

Hypertension forces the heart to work harder and may drive it into failure. It can cause serious injury to the kidneys and progressive impairment of kidney function. It also accelerates the accumulation of fatty deposits in the arteries and substantially increases the risk of heart attacks and strokes.

Among the most important developments of modern medicine are the measures now available to control hypertension. Almost

74

every case, mild or severe, can be treated successfully. In the past decade, the death rate from this cause has been cut almost in half. It can be reduced still further with greater understanding of hypertension.

WHAT IS HYPERTENSION?

Blood pressure is simply the force exerted against the walls of the body's arteries as blood flows through. The force, produced primarily by the pumping action of the heart, is essential for circulating blood and its life-supporting nutrients to all areas of the body.

Each time the heart beats, pressure increases. As we noted in Chapter 2, this upper pressure is called the systolic pressure ("systolic" from the Greek word for contraction), and the pressure at its lowest point, when the heart relaxes between beats, is called the diastolic pressure (from the Greek word for expansion).

To refresh your memory, the normal systolic pressure of a person at rest is in the range of 100 to 140, and the normal diastolic 60 to 90, and a blood pressure reading is expressed by both figures, with systolic over the diastolic: 140/90.

There is, then, a wide span for healthy people. Furthermore, blood pressure normally varies at different times of day and under different circumstances. It is lower during sleep, goes up during physical exertion or emotional excitement.

So a single reading above 140/90 does not indicate abnormal pressure. But when the pressure is continuously elevated, a person is considered to have hypertension.

As we have indicated, hypertension is stealthy. It is easy enough for a physician to uncover it but not for a patient to realize he has it. Mild elevations—and often even severe ones—may produce no symptoms at all. Even when hypertension does lead to symptoms—such as headaches, dizziness, fatigue, weakness—they may not be recognized as being related to the elevated pressure because they are symptoms common to many other disorders.

HOW DOES HYPERTENSION AFFECT
   THE HEART?

First of all, pressure becomes elevated because there is resistance to the flow of blood in the small arteries (the arterioles).
As the heart responds by pumping harder to get the blood through,
pressure goes up. To keep pumping harder, the heart muscle
thickens and dilates—just as when you exercise any muscle
strenuously, the muscle's girth increases. When a muscle increases
in size, it needs increased blood supply. With a great increase in
heart-muscle size, its needs may outpace its supply.

Secondly, hypertension accelerates the development of hardening of the arteries. In any pumping system, wear on both the
pump and pipelines depends on the strain they undergo. If, for
example, a system has been designed to withstand a strain of 100
pounds, it will last longer if the strain never reaches 100 pounds.
If the strain persistently exceeds 100 pounds, the system will
wear out faster. After years of elevated blood pressure, the arteries
may become hardened and less elastic. The impact of the blood,
as it is pumped through under high pressure, may damage the
artery walls. Fat deposits then may accumulate more readily on
these damaged areas, narrowing the arteries and reducing their
capacity for transporting blood. People with hypertension are more
likely than others to develop coronary heart disease.

Hypertension also may damage the blood vessels of the kidneys
and thus impair kidney function. As a result of this impairment,
there may be a tendency for excessive amounts of salt and water to
be retained, and this increases the chance that heart failure will
develop.

In heart failure, the heart does not stop. It goes on pumping.
But it is as if the heart says to itself: "I no longer can work as
hard as I have been doing. I stood up to the load for quite a while,
but I am losing my effectiveness." The heart keeps pumping, but
its contractions are no longer as complete. With each contraction,
less blood is pumped. Heart failure is the loss of pumping efficiency.

Less blood supply goes to the muscles of the body, and so there is muscle fatigue. There is less blood supply for the brain, and so the patient may not be able to think as effectively as he once did. With less supply going to the heart muscle itself, there is coronary insufficiency, a further deficit of oxygen for the pump.

And there is a build-up of pressure within the heart. Unable to pump blood with its old efficiency, the heart retains blood instead of pumping it all out. Pressure within the heart increases; the heart dilates and the dilated chambers become reservoirs for still more blood. The pressure is transmitted backward to the lungs, where the effect is to make them retain fluid. And pressure is transmitted further backward from the lungs to the central veins of the body, the veins of the liver and then the lower extremities. The liver becomes congested and enlarged; the legs swell up with fluids; the neck veins become distended.

It is important to detect and treat hypertension early before such changes have taken place, but it is still not too late to act when they have occurred.

Before considering methods of treatment, it is helpful to understand what is known about the causes of hypertension.

THE CAUSES

A key role in the body's system for regulating blood pressure is played by tiny vessels called arterioles, the smallest branches of the body's arterial tree. The arteries which branch off from the aorta end in the arterioles.

Arterioles have muscular walls and can expand and contract. As they expand, resistance to blood flow is decreased and so blood pressure is reduced. As they contract, resistance increases and blood pressure rises. In effect, an arteriole functions like the nozzle on a garden hose. When you narrow the nozzle opening, the pressure of water in the hose goes up. When you increase the size of the nozzle opening, the pressure goes down.

It is through the arterioles that blood flows into body tissues. And the contraction and expansion of the arterioles makes it possible to control the flow of blood into various tissues—in the digestive tract, the muscles and elsewhere—according to the needs of the tissues at various times.

It is when something goes wrong with the arterioles, when the tiny vessels all over the body become too constricted, that hypertension results.

Many mechanisms help to control the arterioles. Impulses from the nervous system play a role. Certain hormones, such as norepinephrine and epinephrine from the adrenal glands are powerful arteriole constrictors.

One of the known causes of hypertension is a tumor of the adrenal gland, called a pheochromocytoma. It is usually benign rather than malignant, but it produces large quantities of the hormones that constrict the small blood vessels; namely, the arterioles.

Kidney disease or an obstruction to normal blood flow in a kidney artery may cause the kidneys to release a substance that leads to the formation of angiotensin, a powerful blood-vessel constricting agent.

Another cause can be coarctation of the aorta (see page 31). Hypertension from this is in part caused by the mechanical obstruction of blood flow in the aorta itself and in part by the interference with blood flow to the kidneys (the arteries to the kidneys leave the aorta past the point of obstruction).

Aldosterone is a hormone of the adrenal glands which promotes the retention of salt and water by the kidneys. When there is excessive retention, the volume of the plasma (the fluid part of the blood) tends to increase, thus raising blood pressure. Tumors of the adrenal glands may lead to excess amounts of aldosterone, causing excessive salt and water retention.

When any of the above conditions is found to be responsible for hypertension, it is often curable. Surgery to overcome coarctation of the aorta produces prompt relief of elevated blood pressure. So does surgery to remove adrenal-gland tumors or to correct a kidney artery defect. Effective treatment for kidney disease can restore blood pressure to normal.

But such conditions account for no more than 10 to 15 percent of all causes of hypertension.

ESSENTIAL HYPERTENSION

This is the term used for the 85 to 90 percent of cases for which no cause can be established. While a number of possible factors have come under suspicion, none has been proved guilty beyond doubt.

One possibility is a defect, perhaps inherited, in the arterioles themselves. Another is an abnormal irritability of the nervous system which causes excessive stimulation of the muscles that contract the arterioles. Still another possibility is the presence of some abnormal, as yet unidentified, chemical which circulates in the blood and constricts the arterioles.

A strong family history of essential hypertension is a common finding. If one parent has the problem, there is a 50 percent chance that a child may develop it. If both parents are afflicted, the chance increases to 90 percent. This, of course, suggests that hypertension may be an inherited trait. But families have more in common than the genes which determine heredity. They share food, living conditions and many other environmental influences. And it may be that environmental factors affect susceptibility to hypertension.

Obesity is known to be an aggravating factor if not a prime cause of hypertension. Excessive salt in the diet also may elevate pressure.

Most investigators working in the field believe that no single factor accounts for essential hypertension but rather that it is a multifaceted problem: that it may be triggered by any of a number of influences and may be maintained or aggravated by other influences.

Despite the mystery which still surrounds essential hypertension, it is a condition which today can be controlled effectively in the great majority of cases.

THE DOCTOR'S STUDY OF THE PATIENT

To establish, first, that a patient really does have hypertension is not necessarily a simple matter.

In many patients, a blood-pressure measurement will show elevated pressure. But blood pressure, as we have noted earlier, can vary considerably in an individual under varying circumstances. The very fact that a doctor is taking a pressure reading may induce enough anxiety or nervousness to elevate the pressure.

Like many physicians, we prefer to take blood-pressure measurements in the course of two or three visits before coming to the conclusion that a patient really does have hypertension.

During an examination, the physician may use an ophthalmoscope, an instrument to check on the eyes. It makes visible any damage that may have been done by hypertension to the small vessels, the arterioles, in the retina.

The physician can also check on the size of the heart and changes in the heart. He can feel for what is called a left ventricular impulse, which is an indication that the heart has enlarged because it has had to work against high resistance for some time.

Through his stethoscope, the physician may hear a loud sound in the aortic area as the aortic valve closes; that's because the pressure in the aorta is so great that it snaps the leaflets of the valve shut at high speed. He may hear a murmur related to the turbulent flow of blood in the slightly dilated aorta, and this indicates that the hypertension has been present for a long time. He may use the electrocardiograph and fluoroscopy or chest X ray to get a picture of how much the heart has enlarged.

After establishing that hypertension is present and determining what, if any, damage it has done, the doctor must consider the possibility that it results from a known and curable cause.

As we said, the possibility of finding curable hypertension is not great—at best, 15 percent. The search involves thorough physical examination and the use of X rays, various laboratory procedures and some specialized techniques. These include test doses of various drugs; special tests of blood and urine; special tests to determine the way each of the two kidneys is functioning; special X-ray studies of the kidney arteries.

Such tests may entail considerable expense; they are not entirely free of possible complications. To use them routinely in every patient with hypertension would be impractical and ill-advised. The physician must use the best possible judgment in determining those patients in whom a curable type of hypertension is likely to be found.

TREATING ESSENTIAL HYPERTENSION

Hypertension, especially if it is mild, can sometimes be controlled through diet changes alone. For some overweight people, a reducing diet may produce a desirable fall in blood pressure.

Salt restriction, too, may be helpful. This promotes elimination of excess fluids and helps reduce blood pressure. In the past, about one-third of hypertensive patients could be helped to some extent with very stringent salt restriction. Today, such severe restriction is no longer necessary because of modern drug treatment, but moderate salt restriction is often recommended by physicians as an aid to treatment.

The many drugs which have become available to the physician make it possible now to control hypertension of all degrees of severity. These compounds, which have been developed one after the other since the early 1950's, work in a variety of ways.

In addition to the central nervous system, which we use for conscious control of activities, we have an autonomic nervous system which serves to regulate automatically such functions as heart beat and blood pressure. The autonomic system has two divisions which nicely balance each other. One, the parasympathetic division, acts to slow the heart rate and to relax blood vessels. The other, the sympathetic division, does just the opposite, increasing heart rate and constricting the arterioles to raise blood pressure.

Some of the most useful modern drugs act on the sympathetic system, reducing the flow of nervous impulses through it and preventing excessive constriction of the arterioles, thereby reducing blood pressure.

Prior to the availability of these drugs, severe hypertension sometimes was treated by surgery in which the sympathetic nerves were severed. The drugs, in effect, perform a kind of chemical surgery. Furthermore, they often permit more precise control of blood pressure than surgery did, and their effects can be stopped at any time.

Because it may be helpful for you to know about the various types of drugs, let us take a brief look at them.

The Blockers

Among the first effective drugs for hypertension were powerful agents called ganglionic blockers. Nerve systems in the body are not unlike complex home or industrial wiring systems. Nerves branch; they go into the equivalents of junction boxes; other nerves pick up from there.

The sympathetic nerve pathways branch off the spinal cord at various levels to serve different areas of the body. As they branch off, they enter junction centers called ganglia. In the ganglia are spaces, called synapses. A nerve from the spinal column stops at a synapse. On the other side of the space, there is a nerve leading to distant arterioles. For a nervous impulse to get across the space, a chemical reaction must occur. A kind of chemical messenger service comes into play.

Ganglionic blockers block the messenger service. Actually, nicotine had been known to do exactly this since the turn of the century. But nicotine, in the amounts needed, was too poisonous to be used as an antihypertensive drug.

In 1952, a drug called hexamethonium became the first useful ganglionic blocker. It was valuable for severe hypertension but had limited use because it produced such side effects as blurring of vision and constipation.

Another ganglionic blocker, chlorisondamine, which followed, produced a longer, smoother response with fewer undesirable side effects.

The Relaxers

Almost at the same time that the first ganglionic blockers were being developed, a drug called hydralazine was emerging from the laboratory. It produced a more gradual decrease in blood pressure than did the blockers and had a more prolonged effect, which was desirable. Hydralazine appears to act directly on the muscle walls of the small blood vessels, relaxing them.

Soon afterward came reserpine, a drug purified from the Indian plant, *Rauwolfia serpentina*. Reserpine was the first drug to which the term "tranquilizer" was applied. It has a calming effect in the central nervous system. Through that effect, it may reduce the flow of emotionally induced impulses from the central nervous system into the sympathetic system and in that way help reduce elevated blood pressure.

Reserpine also has another effect. The nerve fibers that reach from the ganglia to the arterioles don't actually touch the arterioles but stop just short. When an impulse reaches the end of a fiber, it releases a chemical, norepinephrine, which is manufactured and stored in the fiber ending. And it is this chemical which carries the message for the arteriole to contract. Reserpine acts to reduce the supply of norepinephrine in the fiber endings, thus reducing the number of constricting impulses to the arterioles and bringing down blood pressure.

Reserpine proved of value for many patients with hypertension. For some, however, apathy was a bothersome side effect of the drug. A semisynthetic reserpine compound, syrosingapine, was developed and found to retain the desirable effects of the natural reserpine while producing fewer and milder side reactions.

The Site-Usurpers

More recently there has come a drug called guanethidine. Like reserpine, it reduces the stores of norepinephrine in the fiber endings. But it goes beyond reserpine by occupying the sites usually filled by norepinephrine. As a result, guanethidine has a more sustained effect, which may last as long as two weeks, and is helpful in smooth regulation of pressure.

Another recently introduced drug is methyl dopa. This compound is related to a material that the body uses to produce norepinephrine, and the resemblance is so great that methyl dopa is able to move into the norepinephrine production plant, replacing the other material. Then, what is produced is a kind of counterfeit norepinephrine called alpha methyl norepinephrine. When this is released by a nervous impulse, it is not so effective in passing along the signal to constrict the arteriole, and so blood pressure is reduced.

The Diuretics

Late in the 1950's, a new class of agents called thiazides was discovered. They were to become fundamental to the management of hypertension.

The thiazides are derived from the sulfa drugs often used to combat bacterial infections. Instead of being germ fighters, however, they are diuretics—agents which increase the kidneys' excretion of salt and reduce the retention of fluids. They lower blood pressure. Hydrochlorothiazide is one; there are others. They may be used alone in some cases. In others, they are used in combination with other antihypertensive drugs to bring down pressure effectively. In combination, the thiazides make it possible to use smaller amounts of the other drugs and so reduce the likelihood of side effects.

There are still other drugs as well from which your doctor can choose.

THE RESULTS OF TREATMENT

The value of treatment for even the most severe forms of hypertension has been demonstrated dramatically. Malignant hypertension is a rapidly progressive type of high blood pressure which once killed 80 percent of its victims within a year after it was diagnosed. Now most patients with malignant hypertension can expect effective control.

Other severe types of hypertension are being controlled effectively, and deaths have been reduced through avoidance of complications. As soaring blood pressure has been reduced, enlarged hearts have returned to normal or near-normal, signs and symptoms of heart failure have improved markedly or even disappeared completely, deterioration of kidneys has been arrested, the threat of strokes has diminished. National mortality rates for hypertensive heart disease have been almost halved thus far and are declining further.

With such results even in the very severe forms of hypertension, many physicians now are convinced that further inroads can be made against hypertension and its consequences. Through early treatment of milder hypertension—treatment before there has been extensive damage—it should be possible to greatly reduce the toll of heart failure, strokes, heart attacks and kidney failure.

HOW YOUR DOCTOR CHOOSES YOUR TREATMENT

Your doctor will consider the degree of hypertension you have and many other factors.

If you are overweight, he may begin by prescribing a diet to bring your weight down. He may suggest lowering your salt intake to a more moderate level. If you happen to be a person who bottles up nervous tensions, he may suggest measures to help release the tensions, including exercise and recreational activities. If your hypertension is mild, he may want to see how these general measures work—and often they work well.

If they do not do the whole job of returning your blood pressure to normal limits after a time—or if it is obvious to him from the beginning that they will not be enough—he will use drug treatment, and the drug treatment will be individualized.

He will work to find the right drug or drug combination for you. He will be guided in this by your blood-pressure level and also by your individual reaction to medication. If, for example, a drug is effective for you but tends to make you drowsy, it may be that a reduced dosage will still be effective and not cause drowsiness. Or it may be that a small amount of that drug in combination with small amounts of another drug or of several others will effectively control your blood pressure with minimal or no unwanted effects.

For example, in some cases there may first be a trial of just a sedative such as phenobarbital. Or reserpine may be tried. If either does not help enough, chlorothiazide or a similar diuretic agent may be used. If a diuretic alone does not work well enough, it may be combined with another drug, perhaps hydralazine. If necessary, a third agent such as guanethidine or methyl dopa may be added to the combination.

This may sound formidable, but it isn't really—and it is clearly worthwhile. The objective is to reduce your blood pressure and make you comfortable in the process—to achieve control without penalty.

You can help through your knowledge of the many drugs available and your understanding that no one agent is good for all patients. It will help, too, if you understand that side effects may occur and that you should report these promptly to your doctor so he can evaluate them and try a reduced dosage or a change of medication if necessary.

"A quiet revolution, representing a great unsung victory"—so the medical control of hypertension has been called. The fact is that hypertension is a killer which can now be tamed. And where it is being tamed, it is the result not alone of effective drugs but of cooperation between patient and physician to achieve their most effective use.

If treatment for your hypertension begins when you already have hypertensive heart disease or even when you are suffering from hypertension-induced heart failure, it is still not too late. Your doctor will then add treatment to ease the heart failure. This will involve use of other agents such as digitalis. You will find a discussion of heart failure and its treatment in the next chapter.

We have seen patients hospitalized with severe hypertension, serious hypertensive heart disease and heart failure. Many have been unable to sleep at night or even lie flat because of fluid retention. After a week of intensive therapy, fluid retention has been greatly reduced. Soon thereafter, the heart has begun to decrease in size, and its efficiency has risen enough for them to be able to do simple exercises.

One patient, a thirty-four-year-old woman, had a blood pressure of 260/140. Her heart was enlarged; her neck veins were distended; her ankles were swollen with fluid; she was unable to walk to the bathroom because of shortness of breath. When her blood pressure was brought down to 160/90 with a combination of three drugs and she received digitalis for her heart failure, she lost 60 pounds in three weeks (most of it excess fluid), her heart size decreased and her shortness of breath disappeared. She is now free of marked disability, does her household chores, goes out shopping, and can walk up several flights of stairs.

TO PROTECT YOURSELF FROM HIDDEN HYPERTENSION

If you are free of high blood pressure now, what can you do to protect yourself?

Because hypertension can develop without warning symptoms and may even cause damage of heart, arteries or kidneys without making its presence known, regular physical examinations are essential. They can assure early detection of hypertension and treatment before any damage is done.

There are precautions you can take, too, to minimize the likelihood that hypertension will develop:

1. Keep your weight down. If you were in good health in your early twenties, what you weighed then probably is your ideal weight for a lifetime. Maintain that weight.

2. Eliminate cigarette smoking. When you inhale a cigarette, blood pressure goes up.

3. Keep salt intake moderate. Some studies indicate that a healthy man, for example, needs only ¼ gram of salt a day; but the average American eats almost 10 grams of salt a day, forty times what he needs. Must you really add salt at the table? You get all the salt you need in the prepared foods you eat. Soups, meats, frozen foods, even breads contain it.

[7]

Congestive Heart Failure

Congestive heart failure is not a disease in itself but rather a constellation of symptoms arising from other heart problems. Rheumatic heart disease, hypertensive heart disease, heart infections, heart attacks and many other heart problems can cause it.

As we noted in Chapter 6, heart failure does not represent a final stage of heart disease, but means instead that the pumping performance of the heart has been impaired, that the heart muscle has been so weakened that it cannot provide adequate circulation for body tissues.

The heart normally has a great reserve of power. When you are at rest, your healthy heart uses, on the average, only one-fourth of its maximum power. When you exercise strenuously and your muscles and other tissues have greatly increased needs for oxygen, the healthy heart can therefore quadruple its effort if necessary.

Healthy hearts adapt to the needs of their owners. The heart of a physical laborer or an athlete, for example, is heavier and thicker than the heart of an office worker. Quite normally, the muscle fibers of the heart increase in size to meet the needs of individuals who do heavy work.

Actually, the demands placed on the heart by a heavy worker or athlete are not excessive. For a sedentary person who engages in some activity over a twenty-four-hour period, the work load on the heart may average 150 percent of the base, or lowest, resting work load. A laborer who does heavy physical work may impose an average 200 percent work load on the heart over a twenty-four-hour period, since he is not, after all, working all the time.

But when there is an abnormal condition which affects the heart, the work load can be far greater. For example, if blood pressure is doubled, the basic work load of the heart is doubled— and it is doubled twenty-four hours a day.

Faced with extra demands because of hypertension, heart infection or other abnormal stress, the heart accommodates. It increases in size and weight, and the increase may be much more pronounced than that for a healthy laborer or athlete.

At first the heart does well. It carries the load. To use the medical term, it compensates. It may continue to do so for months, years, sometimes even for a lifetime.

But often, sooner or later, heart failure develops. The muscle fibers have, in effect, become overextended, and they lose strength, somewhat as an overstretched spring does.

The left ventricle loses some of its contracting efficiency. With each contraction, it pumps some blood into the aorta but some blood remains behind. The left atrium has to work harder to move blood into the enlarged left ventricle. Pressure within both the atrium and ventricle increases. After a time, the atrium responds to the pressure by dilating and it, too, accumulates an excess of blood.

The increased pressure in the left atrium is transmitted to the pulmonary vein, which empties blood from the lungs into the atrium, and so the blood flow in the pulmonary vein is slowed and excess amounts of blood begin to accumulate in the lungs. The lungs become heavier and stiffer, and the patient experiences shortness of breath. With the lungs congested, the patient coughs up foamy sputum. And with the congestion, too, fluid may ooze into the space between the lungs and the chest wall, interfering with normal expansion of the lungs.

Meanwhile, the failing left ventricle's inability to pump adequate blood shortchanges the kidneys. As kidney function becomes impaired, urine output drops; not enough water is removed from the blood by the kidneys. The retention of water increases the volume of circulating blood and adds to the congestion in the lungs.

With all this going on, the right ventricle, too, may stretch. The right atrium then has to work harder to fill the enlarged ventricle, thus increasing pressure in the atrium, which is transmitted backward through the vein system. The increased pressure in the vein system interferes with return of used blood from the tissues. Fluid accumulates in tissue spaces, swelling the ankles and the abdomen.

In advanced heart failure, the patient is almost drowning in his own fluids. And the fluid accumulations add to the heart's work, aggravating the failure.

The diagnosis of advanced heart failure can be made by the skilled physician with just a glance at the patient: his neck veins will be distended, his abdomen will protrude and he will gasp for breath.

Diagnosis of early heart failure is not so simple. But the physician is aided by the patient's report of such symptoms as inability to sleep well, mild shortness of breath, some loss of stamina and seemingly inexplicable weight gain. The diagnosis can be confirmed through changes in heart sounds, appearance of lung congestion on chest X rays and laboratory tests.

TREATMENT

The treatment of congestive heart failure is directed at improving the heart's efficiency, eliminating the excess fluids and reducing the overload on the heart. To reduce the overload may require treatment for hypertension or heart infection, or perhaps surgical correction for a defective heart valve if that is the cause. If the main cause is one that cannot be corrected, it is sometimes possible to help the patient by correcting contributing conditions, such as overweight or anemia.

Rest

This is an important element in treatment since it helps to reduce the work load of the heart. The degree of rest required will depend on the severity of the heart failure. In some cases, only mild limitation of activity may be needed; in others, strict bed rest for a time or a combination of bed and chair rest.

Digitalis

More than two centuries old, digitalis remains a mainstay in the treatment of heart failure. In Shropshire, England, eighteenth-century patients suffering from heart failure (it was then called dropsy) resorted to drinking an herbal tea when physicians could not help them. After using it over a long enough period, they would lose water and body weight and breathe more easily. It was discovered that the essential ingredient in the herbal tea was digitalis.

Digitalis might be called a tonic for the heart. It strengthens heart muscle fibers and increases the force of contraction so that pumping efficiency improves. It may improve performance enough that the heart functions effectively even if the condition which caused failure cannot be corrected. Successful treatment with digitalis can break the vicious circle of heart failure; it is not uncommon for a patient with advanced failure to respond by losing 20 pounds of fluid from lungs, abdomen and other tissues.

Many digitalis preparations are now available: long-acting, short-acting, oral, injectable. All are satisfactory, and the physician can choose one he believes best suited to the circumstances. Digitalis is used first in a dose that achieves its full effect and then in smaller daily maintenance doses.

Like other potent medications, digitalis can be toxic in excessive doses. Unwanted effects may include disturbances of heart rhythm, nausea, vomiting, diarrhea, loss of appetite, blurring of vision, headache, lethargy, numbness. The proper dosage for the individual must be determined by the physician and then carefully adhered to. With correct dosage of digitalis, a patient with a failing heart may live many years without severe restrictions on activities.

Diet

Reducing the intake of salt is the chief dietary measure in heart failure. As we said, however, salt no longer has to be severely restricted, thanks to diuretic drugs (see below). Usually, it is possible for the patient to get along well without special salt-free foods, simply by using regular foods without adding salt during preparation or at table. If patients do not respond adequately to treatment for heart failure, more stringent salt restriction may be used.

Fluid intake does not have to be restricted in most patients. Actually, it is now known that when salt intake is reasonably limited, an adequate intake of water and other fluids helps the body keep down salt levels. Moreover, patients allowed normal amounts of fluids are often more comfortable than patients for whom fluids have been restricted. There are exceptions, however, and water restriction sometimes is necessary.

When heart failure is severe, the patient usually tolerates a light diet better than a regular one, and for a time a soft diet may be used. For overweight patients, a diet restricting caloric intake is advisable.

Diuretics

Diuretic drugs, which rid the body of excess fluids, serve a valuable purpose. They make the patient more comfortable; they also reduce the heart load.

Many diuretics are available. In addition to the thiazides, the oral diuretics which are usually taken four times a day, there are powerful mercurial diuretics which are given by injection. Other diuretics, called phthalimidines, have prolonged action and may need to be used only three times a week. And there are still other diuretics which the physician may prescribe as needed.

Mechanical Treatment

Almost always, fluid retention responds at least to some extent to diuretic and dietary treatment. Often the response is entirely satisfactory. When it is not, and when retained fluid in the abdominal and chest cavities makes breathing difficult, the fluid can be removed by needle. And after removal of some fluid this way, not only is the patient immediately more comfortable but there is often an improvement in the response to diuretic treatment.

Other Measures

There are many supportive measures that the physician can use to help the patient with heart failure.

Oxygen is helpful when so much fluid has collected in the lungs that the patient has difficulty getting enough oxygen out of the air he breathes. Oxygen may be administered in a tent or by mask or nasal tube.

Morphine is sometimes useful when breathing is labored. The drug slows the breathing rate so that the patient may breathe more deeply and effectively.

Most patients with congestive heart failure find that they are more comfortable in a reclining or sitting position than they would be if they were lying flat. For others, the physician may find a different position which increases comfort. Until fluid retention is overcome, the physician may recommend that the patient sit up in bed or in a comfortable chair, with legs hanging down so that the blood will tend to pool in the legs. This may increase oozing of fluid from the blood into the tissues of the legs and thus reduce the amount of oozing into the lungs.

In some cases, the physician may find it advisable to use radioactive iodine, which, when taken like a cocktail, reduces the activity of the thyroid gland. A reduction in thyroid activity slows the body's metabolic rate—the rate at which it uses up energy. This, in turn, means that the heart does not have to work so hard, and the patient may improve.

Once, heart failure had to be regarded as an ominous matter. Today, most patients respond well to treatment. Within a few days, they lose weight and fluid, develop increased exercise tolerance and feel much better.

After heart failure has been overcome, proper care can help to assure that it will not recur. What constitutes such care will vary with individual patients. It may include continued use of small doses of digitalis to maintain the strength of the heart. Other medication may be required—perhaps to control hypertension. Attention to diet, particularly to salt intake, may be needed.

With these or other measures the patient who has had heart failure can expect to live many years and to enjoy a productive and reasonably active life.

[8]

Pregnancy and Heart Disease

About 2 percent of all pregnancies in this country are among women who have some form of heart disease. In about 80 percent, it is rheumatic heart disease; in the remainder, hypertensive or congenital heart disease.

The encouraging fact is that today most young women with heart conditions who wish to have children *can* have them safely with the help of good medical management. This is so even though pregnancy increases the work load for the heart.

PREGNANCY AND THE HEART WORK LOAD

Extensive changes in the heart and circulatory system take place as a result of pregnancy—normal changes caused by the fact that the mother's circulation must provide sufficient oxygen and nutrition for both her own body and that of her baby.

The baby's circulatory system develops early. By about the fourth week of pregnancy the fetal heart is beating and blood is circulating. The circulation in the baby is much the same as in

95

an adult, but the baby must depend on the mother for oxygen and food until birth.

The baby's umbilical cord, a cord of tissue and blood vessels, is connected to an organ in the mother's uterus called the placenta. The mother and baby have separate circulations. The placenta is the intermediary between the two. Here, food and oxygen from the mother's circulation are passed along to the baby's circulation, and wastes from the baby's circulation are transferred to the mother's circulation for elimination.

The mother's blood volume increases by as much as 50 percent with pregnancy. Her heart rate increases, too, and reaches a peak of about ten beats per minute over the prepregnancy rate. There is also an increase in the stroke volume; with each beat, the heart contracts more completely and ejects more blood. As a result of the increased beat and stroke volume, the heart output rises by as much as 50 percent.

The burden of pregnancy on the heart and circulation is similar to that caused by vigorous physical exercise but differs in that it is present twenty-four hours a day.

Actually, the burden reaches a peak at the thirty-second to thirty-fourth week. It diminishes in the last few weeks of pregnancy, providing a margin of reserve with which to handle the extra demands of labor. During labor, each contraction of the uterus requires an increase in the heart rate, but rarely does the circulatory burden of labor equal the peak burden during pregnancy.

In caring for a pregnant woman who has heart disease, the physician is concerned with preventing congestive heart failure, which, as we know, is the loss of pumping efficiency of the heart. There is little risk of it before the fifth month of pregnancy. The risk decreases again toward the end of pregnancy when the heart work load diminishes. So if a mother has not developed any heart failure prior to delivery, she is not likely to develop it then.

Some symptoms not unlike those of congestive heart failure often occur during pregnancy in women with perfectly normal hearts. The body, during pregnancy, tends to retain more salt and fluid than usual. This, coupled with pressure factors associated with carrying the baby, may lead to some accumulation of fluid in the legs and cause swelling (edema). A moderate amount of such swelling late in pregnancy is normal.

As the uterus increases in size, it often presses against the diaphragm, which compresses the lungs. This may cause some shortness of breath during mild exertion or even at rest.

During normal pregnancy, too, harmless heart murmurs may appear. They are related to the increased amount of blood pumped by the heart and are only temporary. Some women with quite normal hearts also experience palpitations, or skipped beats.

The physician takes into account such normal phenomena in determining whether a woman with a heart problem is beginning to develop heart failure.

THE RISKS FOR THE HEART PATIENT

Pregnancy, then, is usually well tolerated by a woman with heart disease unless her disease is severe. But some heart patients will be discouraged from having babies. If advanced rheumatic valvular disease or a severe form of congenital heart disease is already taxing the heart's capabilities, leaving little or no margin of reserve, it would not be wise to add as much as 50 percent more work load.

In advising a patient about the wisdom of undertaking pregnancy, the physician must consider the state of her heart and whether it has the capability of taking on the additional burden. The decision may be a complex one requiring the judgment of both obstetrician and heart specialist.

It is important to understand that while pregnancy adds to the work load of the heart, it does not influence the *course* of the heart disease. Heart disease practically never becomes worse because of childbearing if a woman follows her physician's instructions carefully. Life may be shortened, however, if heart failure develops and complicates one or more pregnancies.

The death rate among pregnant women with heart disease is 1 to 2 percent. This compares with a rate of about 0.1 percent for pregnant women who do not have heart conditions. But it must be remembered that the death rate for nonpregnant women with heart disease is higher than for those without such disease.

The fact is, too, that the 1 to 2 percent death rate among pregnant women with heart disease is an overall rate. The risk for a woman who receives continuous medical supervision during her pregnancy can be much less. And she has a better than 90 percent chance of completing her pregnancy and bearing a healthy, living child

RHEUMATIC HEART DISEASE

Rheumatic heart disease is the most common form of heart disease in young women, but fortunately a woman who has it can undertake pregnancy and carry it to a successful conclusio- in most cases.

A history of rheumatic fever also will not stand in the way of most pregnancies. If a pregnant woman has had an attack and is now taking prophylactic medication—penicillin or a sulfa drug —regularly, the medication will cause no harm to her baby and she should keep on taking it.

If rheumatic fever has affected a heart valve, should she have an operation to repair the damage? The answer may well be no, since an operation is not always necessary or desirable. Her physician may advise that she can and should have the baby without surgery.

If an operation is needed, the best time to have it is before a patient becomes pregnant, although operations have been carried out successfully during pregnancy, especially early in pregnancy.

CONGENITAL HEART DEFECTS

Today, more and more young women with congenital heart defects are having babies successfully. This is the result not only of advances in heart surgery but also of increased knowledge about how to care effectively for pregnant women with heart problems.

Congenital heart defects, as we have seen in Chapter 3, are malformations of the heart or great vessels near the heart. A congenital defect may be so slight that it causes no trouble during a long lifetime or severe enough to make the heart incapable of supplying adequate circulation.

As we have seen, too, many of the defects can now be corrected completely; a woman cured of her defect can expect a normal pregnancy. And most women with even partial correction of congenital defects can expect to have children without difficulty.

Congenital defects for which correction is not yet possible may, if mild enough, allow having children. But if a defect produces cyanosis—blueness of blood in the arteries for lack of sufficient oxygen—careful study is needed before the physician can determine whether pregnancy is advisable.

HYPERTENSION

Hypertension comprises 10 to 15 percent of heart disease in pregnancy. If it is mild to moderate and has produced no complications, such as damage to the heart, arteries or kidneys —and the chances are good that it has not produced such complications in a young woman—it is not usually a serious obstacle to pregnancy.

Not only does hypertension not have to bar pregnancy; the reassuring fact is that pregnancy need not worsen the hypertension.

TREATING HEART DISEASE IN PREGNANCY

In ministering to the pregnant patient with heart disease, a major aim of the physician is to keep the total stress on the heart within bounds and leave no opportunity for heart failure to develop.

As we said, extra work for the heart is inevitable, a normal part of pregnancy. But other stress can be reduced. There are many ways this can be done. Excessive physical activity can be avoided. And if obesity is present, weight reduction is helpful.

Any anemia must be corrected, since anemia increases the work load of the heart. The most common type of anemia—iron-deficiency anemia—means that there is a shortage of the iron required for hemoglobin, the substance in blood which carries oxygen. As a result of such anemia, a given amount of blood transports less oxygen from the lungs to body tissues, and so the heart must pump more blood to try to make up for the deficiency. Anemia is usually corrected by a supply of iron either in tablets or in injection.

Excessive functioning of the thyroid (hyperthyroidism), if present, speeds up body metabolism and in so doing places extra demands on the heart. The thyroid gland can be throttled down with radioactive iodine or other treatment.

Excessive salt intake, which promotes retention of fluids and adds to the heart burden, can be avoided.

Any infections—respiratory, urinary or others—which develop can be treated promptly to minimize the strain they impose.

Extra bed rest may be prescribed—two or three hours in the afternoon in addition to at least eight hours of sleep at night.

With such measures, heart failure can very often be avoided, enabling even some women with advanced heart disease to bear children. If these measures do not suffice, others—including treatment with digitalis to strengthen the heart and diuretics to eliminate excessive fluid accumulations (see Chapter 7)—are usually effective. In only rare instances is it necessary today to interrupt pregnancy by abortion because of serious, life-threatening heart failure.

Successful surgery has been carried out during pregnancy for mitral-valve disease and also for some congenital disorders such as patent ductus arteriosus, coarctation of the aorta and pulmonary valvular stenosis. Patients with septal defects do surprisingly well in pregnancy without surgery.

Actually, a recently published study underscores the fact that pregnant women who must undergo open-heart surgery run no greater risk than nonpregnant women—and even stand about a

70 percent chance of having their babies saved. The study covers ten years' experience of twenty heart surgeons with women ranging in age from nineteen to forty-three years and from two weeks to five months pregnant when surgery was performed to correct congenital or rheumatic heart defects. Overall, the death rate as the result of surgery was 5 percent; actually, among patients operated on in the last five years covered by the study, when experience with open-heart surgery was greater, the rate was cut to virtually zero.

Because of the increasing safety of open-heart surgery and the chance of saving such a large percentage of the babies, many physicians now believe that in cases when a heart defect is potentially correctable by surgery but not by medication, the operation should be tried to avoid the need for abortion.

We have had many patients come through such surgery well. Among them was a thirty-two-year-old woman whose pregnancy was endangered during the fourth month by severe mitral stenosis. After an operation to open the mitral valve, she went on to deliver a normal child without difficulty.

When another patient developed severe congestive failure during the fourth month of pregnancy because of mitral stenosis and failed to respond adequately to treatment at home during the next month, it became necessary to hospitalize and confine her to complete bed rest. Oxygen therapy was used for four months before delivery, to help control the heart failure. The woman gave birth to a normal, healthy child and since delivery has been doing well.

Happily, then, most patients today, especially if they seek medical advice before pregnancy and follow that advice conscientiously throughout, can expect to do well and to deliver normal children—and to have a heart none the worse for the experience.

SOME IMPORTANT QUESTIONS AND ANSWERS

How soon should you see a doctor after becoming pregnant? If you know you have heart disease or have had rheumatic fever, see him at once. Better yet, see him before you become pregnant so he can advise you from the start about what you can do to help assure a successful outcome.

Most of the women who have a heart problem and get into serious difficulty during pregnancy are those who seek medical help late and are already in trouble when they seek it.

Make it an absolute rule: if you have been told in the past that you have a heart condition or that you have had rheumatic fever, stay under medical supervision all through your pregnancy. You should have the benefit of good medical care no matter how mild your heart disease or how well you feel.

What advice can the doctor give you before pregnancy? After examining you thoroughly, he can advise you about whether or not you are ready to become pregnant. Probably he will say that you are ready. But if you are not, he may suggest that you build up your general health for a few months by some changes in living habits—in diet, rest, recreation, etc.—before you undertake pregnancy. Or, in some circumstances, he may suggest corrective surgery prior to pregnancy.

If his advice is to go ahead immediately, he can take any steps that may help increase your chances of successful pregnancy —for example, by correcting anemia if it exists, or recommending a diet program to bring your weight to a suitable level.

What is the best diet? Generally, it should be a well-rounded, balanced one. And, generally, that means a varied diet—meats, eggs, poultry, fish, vegetables, fruits, etc., all in moderate quantities.

Specifically, depending on your particular needs, there may have to be caloric restrictions. But it is still essential that the diet remain balanced, and your physician will have definite suggestions about that.

As we've seen, even a woman without heart disease can expect to retain some fluids during pregnancy. Sometimes, especially when heart disease is present, fluid retention can become excessive. Your doctor will keep a close check and if necessary put you on a salt-restricted diet to help eliminate excess fluids.

How often should you see your doctor? A regular schedule of visits is advisable even for a pregnant woman who does not have heart trouble. Your doctor will set one that seems suitable for you and vary it if necessary according to the progress you make.

What symptoms should be considered warnings to contact your physician at once? Swellings of ankles and feet, shortness of breath, palpitations, or skipped beats, and other symptoms occur even in normal pregnancy, and so they are not necessarily related to abnormal heart function. Unless you appreciate this, you may become unduly alarmed. Still, because you do have a heart condition, you should be alert for anything that may signal trouble—and let your doctor decide whether it really does mean trouble.

If you experience morning nausea, which is common early in pregnancy in healthy women, and if it causes repeated vomiting or interferes with your meal-taking, report it to your doctor. Let him know if you cough frequently or cough up any blood, or if you suddenly experience shortness of breath during ordinary housework or other routine activities. Let him know, too, about leg and ankle swellings; let him determine whether your swellings call for treatment.

If you experience a little more fatigue during pregnancy than before, that may mean nothing; it, too, is common in healthy women. But don't hesitate to ask your doctor about it—and certainly report any real exhaustion.

By all means, let your doctor know immediately if you experience a cold, sore throat or fever, no matter how slight. If you have a burning sensation during urination, a possible indication of urinary infection, report it at once. Report, too, any kind of rash.

How will your baby be born? Very likely, by vaginal delivery. Caesarean deliveries are no longer performed simply because a woman has heart disease. There is little likelihood that a woman who has come through pregnancy will have any heart-connected problem during labor and childbirth, for, as we noted, the burden on the heart is less at this point than it was earlier.

Will you pass on your heart disease to your baby? This is not likely. Most heart diseases do not seem to be hereditary. While the cause of most congenital heart defects is not clear—a small percentage seem to result when the mother has German measles early in pregnancy—heredity is not believed to be a factor.

A tendency to develop rheumatic fever may possibly be inherited, but rheumatic fever will not develop unless there is a strep infection.

Can you have many children? Quite possibly, if you wish them. There is no set limit on the number of children for women with heart disease. Each case must be considered individually. It is not solely a question of the burden of pregnancy on the heart. The more young children any mother has, the greater the demands on her, and this is a factor to be considered for the mother with a heart problem. Your physician can give you advice about the number of children you are likely to be able to bear without undue risk—and perhaps, too, about the spacing of pregnancies. Then you and your husband can decide about your family planning.

[9]

Coronary-Artery Disease
and Angina Pectoris

"But there is a disorder of the breast marked with strong and peculiar symptoms. . . . The seat of it, and sense of strangling, and anxiety with which it is attended, may make it not improperly be called angina pectoris. Those who are afflicted with it are seized while they are walking (more especially if it be uphill, and soon after eating) with a painful and most disagreeable sensation in the breast, which seems as if it would extinguish life if it were to increase or continue; but the moment they stand still, all this uneasiness vanishes." This classic description of angina pectoris was written by the English physician William Heberden in 1768. *Angina* means choking or suffocating pain; *pectoris* refers to the breast.

But the agonizing discomfort is really a cry of the heart—the heart's protest when its nourishing blood supply is not adequate to allow it to meet the demands placed on it.

The situation is somewhat comparable to what happens with a car that has a fuel line which has corroded inside, become thick with rust deposits so that its bore is reduced. Enough fuel may flow through the line from the gas tank to the engine for travel at a slow or moderate rate on a level road. But when the driver tries to speed up or there is a hill to be climbed, the fuel flow is inadequate, and the motor sputters because of the inadequacy. So does the heart in angina pectoris.

Angina is not like a heart attack. In a heart attack, blood flow to a part of the heart muscle is suddenly restricted severely or cut off entirely. The particular part of the heart muscle deprived of nourishment is damaged.

Angina represents protest rather than damage. Angina and heart attack do, however, have something important in common: cause. Both usually stem from coronary atherosclerosis, a clogging disease of the coronary arteries which feed the heart muscle.

CORONARY ATHEROSCLEROSIS

As we have seen earlier (Chapter 1), the two coronary arteries that nourish the heart muscle branch off from the aorta, the big trunk artery leading from the heart. The coronary arteries cross along the surface of the heart, giving off a network of branches. Every portion of the heart muscle is supplied with nourishment by this treelike coronary-artery system.

A healthy main coronary artery has a diameter of 2 to 3 millimeters (a millimeter equals $\frac{1}{25}$ of an inch) and will admit a drinking straw. Unfortunately, coronary arteries are affected—have their internal bore decreased—by atherosclerosis. Atherosclerosis may begin to develop early in life, and all of us have it to some degree by the time we reach middle age.

How does atherosclerosis develop? We know the answer from many experiments with animals.

Each coronary artery is made up of an outer cover, middle portion and inner lining. The inner lining, called the intima, consists of several layers.

Blood carries many substances, including lipids, or fatty materials. And the atherosclerosis process starts when cells in the first layer of the intima, for reasons not yet clearly understood, become more permeable to cholesterol and other lipids and allow them to pass through and be deposited within the lining. Each deposit of fatty material is known as an atheroma.

As more and more fat deposits occur, the cells of the lining increase in number and become thickened; calcium from the blood is deposited; and gradually the lining bulges inward, narrowing the channel through which blood flows.

The process is slow, and it does not affect all portions of the coronary arteries equally. Some sections of the arteries may remain unaffected, clear of atherosclerosis; others may be greatly affected.

There are considerable differences in the way coronary atherosclerosis affects people. Many have advanced disease and yet give no evidence of it through a long and active life. They may die at eighty or later from something unrelated to the heart—an accident, an infection, a cancer. They live for a long time, without symptoms of heart disease, because they developed new bypass blood routes—new connections between branches that detour blood around narrowed routes and maintain adequate flow to the heart muscle. On the other hand, many people develop symptoms in their forties and fifties, and some do so even earlier.

THE VARYING SYMPTOMS

At some point as coronary atherosclerosis progresses, there may come the moment when a person experiences his first attack of angina pectoris. It may happen when he is shoveling snow, climbing stairs, playing golf or tennis, or running to catch a bus.

As a rule, as we noted, angina is felt as a constrictive sensation in the midchest, a sensation which often shoots out to the left arm and fingertips. But there are many variations. Occasionally, the pain appears between the shoulder blades, in the left hand or wrist, in the left arm or shoulder, in the pit of the abdomen, in the jaws and teeth, and/or even in portions of the right arm with no chest pain at all. Sometimes, the pain may go from the chest to the elbow or to the fingers. Sometimes, it may start in the arm and then be felt in the chest.

At a recent symposium held at Hahnemann Medical College

and Hospital in Philadelphia, one of our colleagues presented the case of a farmer who felt aching pain in his lower jaw and teeth while walking behind his plow and mule. When he stopped walking, the pain subsided. Since his dentist had found that his teeth were poor, he had them all removed and returned to work with gleaming new false teeth. But again he got pain in his lower jaw while walking behind the plow. He blamed the dentist for not fitting his false teeth properly, and it was only when he consulted a physician that angina was discovered.

Angina, as we have noted, occurs when there is extra demand on the heart which cannot be met because of inadequate supply of blood for the heart muscle. Exercise or other effort may produce an attack. So, very definitely, may emotional stress.

We know, for example, of a banker who likes to play a weekly golf game. It's his major physical activity, and he enjoys it greatly. He feels chest pain when he first addresses the ball to drive it toward the first hole. His "first-hole" angina is related to excitement. He can walk the rest of the golf course, uphill and down, without pain.

One of our colleagues tells of a businessman who loves to hunt birds. He can walk great distances without chest pain, but let him hear the rustle of a flushed covey, and he becomes excited enough to develop angina. Another man loves to gamble: his angina occurs when he holds an unusually good poker hand. As our colleague tells it, "He hurts in his chest when he wins but not while losing. His friends have learned that when he takes nitroglycerin [to control his angina] they dare not raise the bid."

In some cases, angina may occur during sleep. This is called nocturnal angina. Its cause is not completely understood, but it may be the result of dreaming or of irregular heart action.

Usually, an anginal attack compels a patient to stop whatever he is doing. It is not only painful but frightening, awakening a sense of foreboding, of impending doom.

An attack usually lasts only a few minutes. If the pain persists for more than fifteen to twenty minutes, it is not likely to be from angina. The short, extremely disturbing nature of the discomfort is the hallmark of angina pectoris.

The pain stimulus for angina arises in the heart muscle. It is probably caused by noxious chemicals formed there in the absence of adequate oxygen.

While angina is most commonly associated with coronary-artery disease, it sometimes accompanies other heart problems. Angina may occur even though the coronary arteries themselves are healthy if a congenital heart disease or a valve abnormality from rheumatic heart disease interferes with adequate flow of blood into them.

DIAGNOSING ANGINA

Chest pains can stem from many problems which have nothing to do with the heart. The skin over the chest is rich in sensitive nerve endings, and many skin conditions (including shingles, for example) may produce chest pain. Pain from rib fractures and other injuries, from muscular disorders of the chest and shoulder, and from abnormalities of the spine such as osteoarthritis and rheumatoid spondylitis may cause pain that can be confused with angina.

Before arriving at a diagnosis of angina, the physician will take a detailed history including a description—as accurate as the patient can possibly make it—of symptoms and the circumstances under which they occur. He will do a careful physical examination, seeking any evidence of murmurs, rhythm abnormalities or other disturbances which may be associated with heart disease.

The physician may take an electrocardiogram (ECG) while the patient is at rest on a table. If it shows an abnormality indicative of coronary-artery disease, he need go no further. But in more than one-half the patients with angina, the resting ECG is normal, and so if the ECG at rest reveals nothing, another reading is taken after the patient performs a standard exercise such as going up and down a little set of stairs. This exercise ECG is often helpful in diagnosing angina.

When the physician considers them necessary, he may order tests to determine whether there are abnormally increased concentrations of lipids, or fats, in the blood. These would, as we saw, suggest coronary-artery disease.

Another useful means of confirming the presence of true angina is to try the effect of a nitroglycerin pill. In angina, nitroglycerin usually provides relief within five minutes.

RELIEVING ANGINA

The treatment of angina pectoris has several objectives. One is to relieve the pain when it appears. Another is to prevent recurrences. A third is to try to retard or arrest further progression of atherosclerosis in the coronary arteries. And a fourth is to encourage the development of new pathways to feed the heart muscle. If the third and fourth objectives can be achieved, the likelihood of a heart attack is reduced.

Since angina results when the heart is pained by extra demand on it, reducing the demand—stopping exercise or other effort which imposed it—can bring relief. To speed the relief, the physician can prescribe nitroglycerin.

A little tablet of nitroglycerin placed under the tongue and allowed to dissolve there is quickly absorbed into the small blood vessels under the tongue and in seconds is carried by the blood to the coronary arteries.

Nitroglycerin appears to have two effects. It dilates the coronary arteries and perhaps enables them to carry more blood to the heart muscle. It also seems to act on other blood vessels in the body, particularly the arterioles, reducing their resistance to blood flow and easing the work of the heart. Thus, with less work to perform, the heart needs less oxygen; at the same time, oxygen supply is increased because of the improved coronary-artery blood flow.

Nitroglycerin is of course an explosive that burglars use to blow open safes. But it is not explosive in the tiny quantities you take if you have angina.

Unlike morphine and similar drugs, nitroglycerin does not merely "kill" pain. It relieves pain by getting at the cause. You don't develop a tolerance to it so that it loses its effect with time. It provides immediate and striking relief.

Nitroglycerin is a thoroughly tested drug that has been used since 1879. If your doctor prescribes it, take it without hesitation. But make sure that the nitroglycerin is fresh. If it crumbles easily, it should not be used. Heat and light destroy its effectiveness, so it should be kept in a dark bottle and in a cool place. It can be kept in the refrigerator but not in the freezer.

PREVENTING PAIN

If you have angina, your physician will try to minimize the likelihood of repeated attacks. He may do this in many ways.

He will check for high blood pressure, active peptic ulcer, gall-bladder disease, and severe anemia—all of which may impose added stress on the heart—and if any of these are present, he will take steps to correct them, usually through medication and diet.

He will review with you your daily activities to determine which exertions trigger angina episodes. Modification of a patient's routine—often simple modification—can be most helpful. For example, your physician will probably advise you to avoid walking immediately after meals, since the process of digestion adds to the work of the heart and it is unwise to add further to it by walking.

But any physical activities that do not induce chest pain need not be discouraged. And any essential activities which do lead to pain can often be carried out without discomfort if nitroglycerin is taken immediately beforehand. Similarly, if sexual intercourse is followed by angina, nitroglycerin taken beforehand may prevent the pain.

Nitroglycerin *should* be used prophylactically in anticipation of events that are generally followed by angina. If nitroglycerin taken before setting out in the morning, before playing a first hole of golf, before walking up a hill or before moving the bowels can prevent discomfort, it is all to the good to take it. There can be no possible harm if nitroglycerin is used this way in the dosage your physician prescribes

Too many patients do not use nitroglycerin prophylactically. They are aware of its benefit when an angina attack occurs, but they wait until the attack before using the medication. They seem to feel that it is better to avoid use of nitroglycerin if at all possible. Such patients need to be reassured about the safety of using nitroglycerin and the importance of taking it both with initial symptoms of angina rather than the peak pain and also beforehand, prophylactically, when they know that some necessary activity or situation is going to provoke an attack.

It is certainly wise for the person with angina to learn to avoid undue excitement as much as possible. Anxiety may be alleviated, when necessary, by barbiturates or tranquilizing drugs prescribed by a physician.

If a patient is overweight, his physician will suggest an appropriate diet. By reducing, he spares the heart the extra work of pumping blood to nourish needless fat. And reducing provides another benefit for the heart, for the less weight the muscles and other structures have to support, the less blood supply *they* need.

As a demonstration of the wisdom of getting rid of excess weight, some physicians ask a patient, during an office visit, to lift a medical instrument that may weigh 15 or 20 pounds and then walk around the office or down the hall with it. The patient quickly appreciates the burden of the excess weight he is carrying around at all times.

DIETING

Even if you are not overweight, your physician will very likely have advice for you about diet as a means of trying to halt or at least retard atherosclerosis. And if you are overweight, the reducing diet he suggests will take this into account, too.

As you will see in Chapter 14 on preventive measures, certain types of foods high in saturated fatty acids appear to play a role in atherosclerosis. In place of them, your physician may suggest foods with fats high in unsaturated fatty acids.

Your physician will make certain that a weight-reducing diet, if it is necessary, will be healthy for you not only in terms of the atherosclerosis but also in terms of the general needs of the body. The diet will contain a suitable mix of proteins, carbohydrates and fats to provide all essential elements, including vitamins and minerals.

It is a mistake for anyone to indulge in fad reducing diets— and it is a serious mistake for a person with coronary-artery disease and angina to do so.

Your physician may suggest that instead of eating three standard meals a day, you eat five or six smaller ones. Each is easier to digest and requires less heart effort. Many people find, too, that smaller, more frequent meals help in taking off and keeping off excess weight.

Usually coffee and tea are permitted in moderation unless they cause abnormal heart rhythms or chest pain or interfere with sleep. While there is no solid evidence that alcohol is beneficial to the coronary-artery circulation, it may have some value through its relaxing effect.

Along with diet, there are now some medications which give promise of helping to reduce the levels of cholesterol and other fatty materials in the blood. They are not invariably necessary, but your physician may decide that use of one in your case is indicated. We will discuss these medications in Chapter 14, too.

OPENING UP NEW BLOOD PATHWAYS

As we have seen, nature has endowed the heart with a remarkably adaptable coronary-artery system. When one coronary artery becomes narrowed, branches from the other coronary artery may take over some of the job of getting blood to an affected area of the heart muscle.

Since the coronary system has the capacity to form new branch vessels and connections—called collateral circulation—some people with severe coronary atherosclerosis never experience angina or have a heart attack. For them, collateral-circulation formation keeps pace with the atherosclerotic process. As some narrowing takes place, some collateral circulation develops; as the narrowing increases, so does the collateral-circulation formation. Because the two processes dovetail, at no time is there any serious circulation deficit for the heart.

In the patient with angina, this obviously has not been true. Collateral circulation formation has lagged behind the advance of atherosclerosis. Still, it may not be too late to change the picture—not only with diet and drugs but by stimulating collateral-circulation formation.

For such stimulation, it is essential that the patient avoid becoming an invalid and instead make moderate, well-adjusted demands on the heart.

Although the idea of exercise for a patient with angina may seem irrational, many physicians have long felt it could be helpful. If started slowly and built up gradually, always stopping short of the point of provoking angina—and patients are often able to discern at what point chest pain will develop—such activity can stimulate the development of collateral circulation.

Many physicians have learned about exercise from their angina patients. They have seen, for example, a patient with a great love of golf refuse to give up the game after becoming a victim of angina. He may have been able to play only a hole or two and at a very slow pace in the beginning. But by persisting, he gradually reached the point of being able to play 18 holes without difficulty and to carry over his increased exercise tolerance into regular daily activities.

Recently, there have been many studies aimed at trying to measure objectively the results of carefully designed exercise programs. They indicate that some patients do benefit, with increased exercise tolerance and reduction of anginal symptoms.

Studies are continuing to learn in detail about the usefulness of physical reconditioning, how it may best be employed and for which patients.

It should be obvious that a patient should not undertake an exercise program on his own. Excessive exercise can precipitate a heart attack. Exercise should be begun very slowly and carefully, with the approval of the physician, and then increased very gradually under his supervision.

THE OUTLOOK

The prospects are increasingly good today for most patients with angina.

In our past experience, of every hundred patients with angina, about seventy-five could expect to live five years; about sixty, ten years; and about forty, fifteen years or longer. These were overall expectancies covering all degrees of severity of angina and underlying disease.

Today, the outlook is better—and particularly so when the angina and underlying disease are not far advanced when treatment is sought. There is a new attitude of optimism in the medical profession. There are added tools to work with, expanding knowledge.

There are methods, too, for bringing under control even very severe, seemingly intractable, angina.

The term *intractable angina pectoris* implies a hopeless state, a point of no return—and yet many patients can now be helped.

In intractable angina, the patient usually has frequent episodes of pain triggered by slight exertion or mild emotional stress. Sometimes the episodes occur when the patient is at rest. Intractable angina may develop when the atherosclerotic disease process is outdistancing collateral-circulation development.

When this happens, there are many measures that can be used. Often, a period of hospitalization brings relief because the patient is away from daily stresses. Mild sedation can be helpful. A gradual return to routine living then may be possible.

Sometimes seemingly intractable angina proves to be the one overt indication of early congestive heart failure. In that case, the angina can be relieved with digitalis or other appropriate treatment for the heart failure.

In other instances, seemingly intractable angina may be the result of abnormal heart rhythms. If so, medication to prevent those rhythms will help overcome the angina problem.

Some seemingly intractable cases of angina improve when the patient can be convinced of the value of paying stricter attention to diet, to lighter and more frequent meals, to prophylactic use of nitroglycerin.

It is a fact, too, that when angina seems to be intractable, other causes may be involved. Duodenal ulcer, diaphragmatic hernia, local chest-wall tenderness, tendonitis, bursitis or other problems sometimes simulate angina; they may also exist along with angina and at times trigger it. Treatment of these conditions may reduce the frequency of anginal attacks.

When angina fails to yield to other measures, radioactive iodine may be used to reduce the activity of the thyroid gland. This helps reduce the heart's work and may reduce the angina episodes.

SURGERY FOR ANGINA

Over a period of many years, there have been efforts to develop surgical procedures for overcoming severe angina by increasing the supply of blood to the heart muscle.

Some of the more recently developed procedures appear to be promising. They are discussed in Chapter 16.

[10]

The Heart Attack

The place can be any American community. The time: shortly before midnight. In a bedroom of a quiet, darkened home, Mr. Jones, a man in his early fifties, wakes to a sense of uneasiness. He had had a long, hard day, had eaten a hearty dinner and had retired early.

As he shifts in bed, he becomes more aware of a feeling of heavy pressure under his breastbone. Indigestion? In the bathroom, he mixes a solution of bicarbonate of soda and drinks it.

His wife is up now, inquiring. "Just indigestion," he tells her. But as he sits down on the edge of the bed, the pain in his chest is worse, and he is perspiring profusely, feeling faint and short of breath. And when Mrs. Jones picks up a telephone and calls the doctor and tells him that she thinks her husband is having a heart attack, Mr. Jones offers no protest.

When the doctor arrives, he gives Mr. Jones a morphine injection to relieve the pain. The first injection helps very little, and he repeats the injection to better results. Mr. Jones is moved to the hospital. Oxygen is administered.

There are electrocardiogram and other tests. The chest pain

117

continues to be great enough to require morphine injections. It decreases on the second day. But Mr. Jones has fever now which persists for four days.

When the fever leaves, he feels well. But he has to remain in the hospital for another three weeks—so that, as his doctor tells him, the damaged heart has a chance to heal more completely.

For part of that time, he remains in bed. While in bed, he does gentle leg and foot exercises frequently to avoid the pooling of blood in his leg veins. He feeds himself, and the meals are kept small to reduce the work demand on the heart that digesting heavy meals entails. He loses weight—and that is to the good.

Soon he is encouraged to sit on the edge of his bed for a few minutes several times a day. Not long after that he is sitting up in a chair for short, then increasingly longer, periods. Two weeks after his heart attack, he is allowed to have friends visit him and then business associates.

Four weeks after his admission to the hospital, Mr. Jones goes home, feeling weak but otherwise well. He is encouraged to walk about at home and even to climb stairs (slowly).

Ten weeks after his attack, he is back at work. He has lost 15 pounds, has not smoked cigarettes since the day of his attack and now feels, he says and means, better than he has felt in years.

A recovery such as Mr. Jones has made is far from rare. Many, many thousands of people each year make similar recoveries from a heart attack—or, as doctors call it, coronary occlusion with myocardial infarction. Coronary occlusion means that a coronary artery has been closed off. Myocardial infarction means that a part of the heart muscle (myocardium) has died (infarction) because the artery closure caused it to lose its normal supply of oxygenated blood.

Heart attacks do not always produce the same symptoms. Very severe pain in the chest will sometimes spread into the throat, the shoulders, the arms and even the back. In addition, there can be nausea and vomiting, sweating and sudden intense shortness of breath.

But the classic hallmark of a heart attack is chest pain. It may range from a slight feeling of pressure to the feeling that the chest is being crushed in a vise. Some people are immediately prostrated; others walk about trying to find relief.

The patient who suffers a heart attack after having had angina may assume at first that this is angina again. But this time nitroglycerin does no good. Nor does stopping activity help, as it does when the pain is anginal.

Typically, the pain which occurs with a heart attack lasts for several hours and does not subside until a narcotic such as morphine is administered.

Accompanying the pain almost always is a feeling of terrible anxiety, a sense that death is near. Commonly, the face turns ashen gray and there is a cold sweat.

Often, there is retching, belching of gas and vomiting—which is why a heart attack is sometimes confused with a stomach upset.

Shortness of breath is common. With a very severe attack, a patient may gasp and struggle for air as though he had acute asthma. Occasionally, there can be loss of consciousness.

Some patients experience palpitations—sensations that the heart is beating abnormally fast and hard.

But a heart attack can occur with little pain—merely unexplained weakness, sweating or breathlessness. And sometimes an attack comes with no pain at all. It is believed to be painless in as many as 10 percent of the cases. This is a hard statistic to evaluate and may not be valid. In many cases of so-called silent heart attack—in which the finding is made on the basis of electrocardiographic changes—close questioning shows that there was *some* pain which was ignored as inconsequential. There may have been a sharp twinge or two which gave place to a continual dull ache that the patient passed off as not worth serious attention.

Actually, the severity of pain accompanying a heart attack does not necessarily indicate the severity of the attack. People who experience only modest discomfort could nonetheless have a major heart problem—and, conversely, those with severe pain may have only mild damage.

Each year there are some 800,000 new cases of coronary occlusion and myocardial infarction in this country. Four of every seven persons suffering the first heart attack survive the attack. The survival rate is even greater for mild, uncomplicated heart attacks; that rate reaches 95 percent. Because of the magnificent vitality and adaptability of the human heart, the survivors often lead long and virtually normal lives.

Overall, without regard to how serious the attack was, about two-thirds of heart-attack patients are alive at the end of five years; about half are alive at the end of ten years. And those who die are, for the most part, older people, many of whom might not have lived the ten years even if they had never had a heart attack.

These, in effect, are statistics from the past. We are certain that the statistics which will become available five, ten, twenty and more years from now for the survival of patients experiencing heart attacks today will be even more satisfactory. For we know more today about how to reduce the risk of a recurrence of heart attack.

Morbid fear of heart attacks is wasteful. All of us would do better to understand the nature of heart attacks; what can be done to prevent them (we shall discuss this in Chapter 14); and, if a heart attack does occur, what can be done to help the heart repair itself.

HOW IT HAPPENS

Although a heart attack occurs suddenly, it is the result of a slowly developing disease process, atherosclerosis of the coronary arteries, as we have seen in the preceding chapter.

With the slow accumulation of fatty deposits in an artery lining, the passageway for blood flow is narrowed. At the same time it is roughened; scarlike fibrous tissue forms and projects into the blood stream. Blood flowing through may form clots around these projections. If a relatively large clot should form in a narrow artery, it may block the passageway and shut off the flow. The result is a heart attack. A part of the heart ordinarily supplied by that artery no longer receives blood and oxygen. This part of the heart begins to ache, and that is the pain felt in a heart attack.

A heart attack does not necessarily have to occur in the midst of activity, as is typical for angina pectoris. There have been studies indicating that as many as 50 percent of heart attacks occur while people are asleep or resting, and another 20 percent during the most modest type of physical activity.

But unusual exertion can provoke an attack. During severe exertion, pressure within a narrowed coronary artery rises and may lead to bursting of small blood vessels in the artery wall; the bleeding may cause rupture of an atherosclerotic deposit. The material may get into the blood in the coronary artery, be swept along, and may finally block a smaller vessel downstream.

Emotional stress, too, may trigger a heart attack by causing increased secretion of certain chemical substances, called catecholamines. These add to the work of the heart and may also favor development of a clot within a coronary artery.

Occasionally, injury to the chest wall is associated with a heart attack. The injury may cause death to heart muscle tissue directly or may affect a coronary artery and lead to clot formation.

HOW THE HEART RESPONDS

The pain that occurs with a heart attack continues for some hours. During this time, the damaged part of the heart muscle has not yet died; it is still trying to struggle along.

Gradually, however, the fibers of the damaged part of the muscle stop contracting, and swell up and die. As this happens, the pain begins to disappear.

Now healing starts. The process is the same as when other parts of the body are injured. Leukocytes, or white blood cells, are mustered. The leukocytes engulf and remove the dead muscle fibers. The removal is essential if remaining tissue is to heal. The clearing-away process may require a week or a little longer, and during this time there may be slight fever.

At the same time, other repair processes are under way. We talked earlier (see Chapter 9) about collateral circulation, the coronary system's ability to form new branch vessels and connections. The moment a coronary artery is closed off, there is an intensive spur to new collateral formation. New branch vessels develop to bring blood to the area around the injury in the heart muscle, and this augmented blood supply plays an important role in healing.

The dead area of the heart muscle cannot be restored. It is replaced by scar tissue. As healing in the affected heart area takes place, a scar begins to form. It usually builds up within the first two or three weeks after an attack.

It takes time for the scar to become firm and tough. The length of time depends on the extent of the injury and the individual healing rate. Usually a month to six weeks is needed.

There is no word other than miraculous to characterize the arrangements the body makes after a heart attack to heal the damaged area and to create new pathways for adequate blood supply to the area around the injury.

And medicine's role after a heart attack is to do everything possible to give the body an opportunity to make its arrangements and to prevent complications that would interfere.

DIAGNOSIS

Physicians are trained to observe how a patient uses his hand when he describes his pain. If he places his hand across his chest, palm down, with fingers spread, and with the center of the palm located over the center of the chest, and then motions as if he is about to squeeze the whole chest into the confines of his palm, a physician can practically vouch that a true heart attack has occurred.

When it is necessary to resolve any doubts, the physician can resort to tests.

The ECG, as we have noted earlier, records the electrical activity of the heart muscle. When the muscle is injured, there is some change in electrical activity which can be noted on the ECG. When part of the heart muscle dies, the ECG may reflect that fact. Abnormalities on the ECG may be noted as early as thirty minutes after onset of symptoms of a heart attack, but in most patients they do not appear for several hours and in rare instances may be delayed four or five days or longer.

One helpful laboratory test measures the level of certain enzymes in the blood. Normally, the heart muscle contains a higher concentration of many enzymes than does the blood stream. After a heart attack and damage to part of the heart muscle, some enzymes from the damaged area pass into the blood stream, raising the concentration there. One of these enzymes is SGOT (serum glutamic oxaloacetic transaminase). Another is LDH (lactic dehydrogenase). Thus when a test reveals high levels of these enzymes in the blood, the possibility of heart attack is indicated. Since similar enzymes occur in other tissue—the lungs and liver, for example—the test may not be conclusive in itself. Nevertheless, when coupled with the patient's symptoms and other findings, it often corroborates the diagnosis.

Recent work indicates that manganese levels in the blood may provide a valuable confirmatory test for heart attack. Manganese is a mineral present in the heart muscle. After an attack, the heart may release up to 60 percent of its manganese. Manganese levels in the blood begin to rise after eight to ten hours and stay elevated for five to six days.

TREATMENT

One major aim of treatment is to create the most favorable conditions possible for healing of the heart muscle. Another is to encourage the development of collateral blood vessels to get more circulation to the areas around the damaged muscle and to help the undamaged part of the heart muscle carry on. A third is to prevent complications.

Relieving Pain

This is an important first step. Pain relief does more than make the patient comfortable, important as that is. Pain causes spasm or contraction of the coronary arteries; it leads to excess secretions of catecholamines, chemicals which increase heart rate and heart work; it also produces restlessness and excess activity. A patient freed of pain has the chance to get maximum heart rest.

As we have seen, a physician is likely to administer morphine or another narcotic pain-relieving agent immediately, but rarely is it necessary to use narcotics after the first few days following a heart attack. There need be no worry about the patient's becoming a drug addict.

Oxygen

Oxygen is not always needed. If breathing is particularly difficult, it may be used. In some cases, it is needed for only a short time. In others, it may be administered for several days or perhaps a week.

When oxygen is administered—through a mask or nose tube or in a tent—a rich supply gets into the blood and so the supply to the heart muscle is greatly increased. Actually, oxygen often helps to diminish pain in addition to easing labored breathing. It also has the effect of making a patient less restless and aiding sleep.

Rest

Although damaged, the heart must still pump blood through the body. It needs rest but can't have it—not complete rest. But comparative rest is possible and most desirable.

Every movement you make adds to the heart's work, since it uses up oxygen and therefore demands increased blood circulation. Thus, bed rest is an essential part of treatment. In the beginning, the patient may have to permit himself to be fed and bathed to keep his movements and the demands on his heart to a minimum.

Obviously, the more complete the rest, the more all activity is avoided, the greater the ease for the heart. But other factors must be considered. Complete rest is not good for other parts of the body, including muscles and lungs.

There have been changes in the concept of what constitutes effective rest. As recently as the 1940's, the practice often followed involved putting a patient flat in bed, admonishing him to move as little as possible, and spoon-feeding him. Now less restrictive measures are known to be more effective for the patient's heart, comfort and general health.

At some point during the first week after the heart attack, the patient may be encouraged to breathe deeply at regular intervals, to turn from side to side, and to move his legs. Quite possibly, during the first week, too, he may be raised to a sitting position in bed. During the second week, he may be feeding and washing himself. During the fourth week, he may be sitting over the edge of the bed. In the fifth week, he may be using a bedside commode and having meals out of bed.

Actually, if the heart attack has been relatively mild, all this may be speeded up greatly, and he may even start to walk in three weeks or less.

Keeping Calm

Anger, fear and other emotions may seem to be purely matters of feeling. But, in fact, they involve the body; indeed, part of the reason for emotions is to prepare the body for physical action. Probably you can recall times when your heart pounded because of fear. Much else was going on within your body at the same time. With emotion, the body glands pour out more secretions, the muscles become tense, the blood flows faster, you breathe more quickly. You are being readied to fight or flee in the face of some danger or challenging situation.

It is important that, as much as possible after an attack, the heart be spared the extra effort demanded of it by emotional upset. If the patient feels anxiety about his condition, and most patients do after a heart attack, his physician will try to relieve it by encouraging him to bring out in the open the thoughts that are bothering him. Talking out his worries and fears rather than bottling them up is of great value. And the value is increased when, as so very often happens now, the physician can provide reassurance that despite the damage to his heart, he is going to recover and the chances are good that he is not going to be an invalid.

Sedation is used for practically every patient because anxiety is so common. Many stress-relieving agents are now available. In addition to barbiturates and similar agents, there are tranquilizing drugs which may relieve mental tension, anxiety and emotional stress with very little sedation. These drugs serve a useful purpose.

At first, visitors will not be welcomed. Later, when the patient feels well enough to want to see people, the doctor will probably relax the ban, particularly for cheerful, sensible visitors. And to the degree that reading, watching television and listening to the radio do not overexcite, they, too, will be permitted.

Diet

The diet will be planned to place a minimum burden on the heart. Digestion calls for extra heart work. The heavier the meal, the more the work.

In the first few days, the doctor may prescribe only broth, weak tea and fruit juices. Such limited intake helps keep gaseous distention to a minimum, thereby avoiding this burden for the heart as well.

Later the patient will be served light meals designed to provide nourishment and strength—four or five of them instead of less frequent heavy meals.

Anticoagulant Treatment

This may or may not be considered necessary, depending on each condition. Anticoagulants are drugs which help to keep the blood from coagulating or clotting easily. Once a clot has formed, anticoagulants do not reduce its size, but they may prevent additional clot formation.

Preventing and Treating Complications

In many patients, recovery follows a smooth course after a heart attack. But complications do sometimes occur, and the physician is always alert for them.

One is shock. When the heart muscle is injured, arteries distant in the body may respond through a kind of automatic reflex action by becoming excessively dilated. When this happens blood pressure falls and the patient develops pallor, cold and moist skin, and rapid pulse. Shock may develop even when the heart muscle has not been extensively damaged: a patient may have a shock reaction, recover from it, and walk out of the hospital with a heart that is still basically sound.

For the treatment of shock, oxygen and other supportive measures may be used, along with drugs to restore blood pressure. The physician now has many drugs to choose from—among them Aramine, Wyamine, Neo-Synephrine and Vasoxyl. With an effective drug, a rise in pressure occurs within ten minutes. When a drug does not bring pressure up adequately after it is injected into a muscle or under the skin, it may do so if infused into a vein. If the result is still not satisfactory, another more powerful agent such as Levophed may be infused. And if this proves inadequate, a cortisonelike agent may be effective.

Another possible complication is pulmonary edema—accumulation of excess fluids in the lungs. Treatment for this includes administration of oxygen and morphine. Digitalis, too, may be used to strengthen the heart, improve its function and aid circulation so the fluid accumulation is reduced. To prevent recurrence of the edema, a diuretic drug may be used.

Mild congestive heart failure, which is discussed in Chapter 7, is not uncommon in the early days after a heart attack. Rarely does it need intensive treatment. The patient is already at rest. Restriction of salt intake helps; so does use of a diuretic drug. These measures are usually enough.

Another complication is the development of an irregularity of heartbeat, a cardiac arrhythmia. Some irregularities are of little consequence, merely temporary annoyances. But others are of great importance. In fact, in the past serious arrhythmias have probably been the most common cause of death in patients hospitalized for heart attacks.

With a serious arrhythmia, the smooth contraction sequence of the heart is upset. This may lead to fibrillation—irregular and ineffectual motion of the heart. And fibrillation may progress to cardiac arrest—stoppage of the heart.

Even when cardiac arrest occurs, prompt action may save life. The heart may be started again by expert thumping of the chest with a physician's clenched fist, or by external heart massage, or by opening the chest and manipulating the heart manually until it begins to beat again.

Fortunately, when fibrillation is detected, the useless beating can be stopped before it leads to cardiac arrest. A fibrillating heart can be converted into a normally beating heart with a defibrillator, a device that shocks the heart electrically.

And, even more fortunately, we now know which abnormal rhythms precede fibrillation, and prompt treatment for these— with various medications including quinidine and procaine amide —often can prevent it.

The early recognition and treatment of abnormal rhythms— to reduce deaths among heart-attack patients—is a major reason why several thousand hospitals have established special coronary care units (CCU's), and why more and more other hospitals are now setting them up.

In a CCU, a heart patient is under round-the-clock observation in the first days after an attack, when abnormal rhythms are most likely to develop. He is examined frequently by medical personnel, and electronic monitoring equipment continuously records his electrocardiogram, blood pressure, pulse rate and other vital information. The data are displayed on a screen in the patient's room and often, too, at the nursing station.

Any change that might herald the beginning of a serious abnormal rhythm sets off an audiovisual alarm system to summon medical aid. Emergency drugs, defibrillators, and other resuscitation equipment are kept close at hand, often in the patient's own room, so no time is lost in initiating lifesaving measures. Nurses are specially trained so that if a doctor is not immediately available they are capable of starting lifesaving procedures without delay.

CCU's (see Chapter 17 for additional details about them) have produced striking gains. With prompt detection and management of abnormal rhythms, the death rate, overall, of hospitalized heart-attack patients has been cut in half. In some of the longest-established and most experienced CCU's, deaths from heartbeat irregularities have been reduced almost to the vanishing point.

MORE ABOUT HOW YOUR HEART HEALS ITSELF

Aided by good medical care, which provides the favorable conditions and prevents or promptly treats any endangering complications, the heart can often do a remarkable repair job on itself. We mentioned this earlier but, because an understanding of it is so important to any heart-attack patient, we want to go into a little more detail here.

First, try to picture the actual damage. Think of a river which flows hundreds of miles, providing water for many communities along the way—a great river, fed by other rivers as well as by small creeks.

Suppose some catastrophic event of nature blocks the river. From the place of blockage on, every community along the way will suffer. But if the blockage occurs far downstream, only a few communities will be affected. Those upstream will still get their water. And if the blockage occurs in a little creek flowing into the river, hardly anybody may suffer.

As we have indicated earlier, the coronary arteries and their many branches form an intricate network around and through the heart. Theoretically, a clot can lodge almost anywhere in that network and obstruct flow. If it lodges in a main artery or a major branch of a main artery, it is as if the river is blocked high up-stream; much of the heart, as much of the population served by the river, will feel the effects. If, however, as very often happens, the clot blocks only a tiny branch, only a small portion of the heart muscle will suffer.

Another consideration of recovery is *when* the heart attack de-veloped. As we have indicated, while the heart attack is a sudden affair, the underlying process that leads to it is not sudden at all but goes on for a long period. And often, over an extended period of time, with the slow narrowing of an artery and gradual reduc-tion of blood flow, collateral circulation pathways have been de-veloping. They help in the heart's adaptation to a heart attack.

Furthermore, there is perhaps no other organ of the body so capable of making quick additional adaptations in an emergency.

Fever, you will recall, develops soon after a heart attack. A sign of illness? Yes, in one sense. But it is also a sign of healthy activity. It occurs as white blood cells rush to the scene and begin to digest and get rid of the dead tissue which would be only a drag on the heart.

The white cells may also attack the clot, boring through it or liquefying it. Meanwhile, nearby vessels are growing to take on the blood-circulation job; some of these may even grow into the clot mass and help get rid of it. It is thus possible for a blocked artery to become unblocked.

Nor is that all.

Blood is pumped into arteries under pressure. When an artery is blocked, there is no pressure beyond the point of blockage. But nature provides for interconnections between one coronary artery and another through many branches and capillaries. So with blood pressure remaining normal in the unobstructed artery but absent beyond the blocked point in the other artery, blood crosses over, flows readily through branches and capillaries into the obstructed artery beyond the point of obstruction. Thus there is a waiting, built-in detour mechanism to respond to the heart's needs in an emergency.

One might consider this a purely resuscitative mechanism. The obstruction has occurred; the heart has been wounded; detoured blood answers the call. Actually, however, if the obstruction occurs in a minor coronary branch, the detouring blood may get to the small affected heart-muscle portion quickly enough so that there is almost no lasting damage. In fact, sometimes as a result of this mechanism, a patient has a minor heart attack, experiences little or no pain and remains unaware of the event.

If a main artery has been obstructed, the detour mechanism may not be able to get enough of the large amounts of blood needed through in time to prevent serious oxygen deprivation of the heart muscle. But it may still help in limiting the damage and in enabling the heart to go on functioning.

Again, it is the wonderful adaptability of the heart and of the circulatory system that supplies it that makes possible recovery from a heart attack, especially if everything possible is done to take care of or prevent complications.

Once you have recovered from a heart attack, the outlook need not be bleak. Far more often than not, the patient who remains an invalid after a heart attack does so because of misunderstanding and needless fear and anxiety, rather than because of damage to his heart.

[11]

The Return to
Useful Living

The great majority of people who recover from heart attack are able to return to activity; only 10 percent are severely limited in what they can do.

Early in 1963, soon after Lyndon Johnson took over the toughest job in the country, anti-American rioting erupted in the Republic of Panama. Night after night, the new President could get only four hours of sleep—to the alarm of many people concerned over the state of his health. The worry stemmed from the day eight years before when Johnson, then Senate Majority Leader, was struck by a heart attack. How could a victim of heart disease subject himself to such violent physical and mental stress without damaging his health? But nothing happened. Despite all the stresses of his time in office, his heart remained healthy.

When President Dwight Eisenhower suffered a heart attack in 1955, there were conjectures that he might be incapable of serving out the remaining months of his first term; a second term was thought impossible. Again the pessimists were confounded.

The two Presidents are examples of patients who returned to useful living after heart attacks. Newspapers, of course, tell of the people who die of heart attacks; they do not tell of the many thousands who return to families and careers and to life as they liked to live it before—because this is not news.

Physicians, learning more and more about the remarkable intrinsic toughness of the heart and its reserve powers, now often actively encourage "cardiacs" to resume their careers. And the careers aren't necessarily confined to the executive suite, where strain may be mainly mental. On the advice of their doctors, some former heart-attack patients are digging ditches, driving bulldozers, and punching rivets in skyscrapers.

Dr. Irvine H. Page, former president of the American Heart Association, said: "Returning to work won't increase the chance for attack. In fact, if a worker doesn't return to work, the frustration he feels from being treated as an invalid definitely increases the potential for another attack."

Dr. Paul Dudley White, who tended President Eisenhower, says: "I would like to emphasize the fact that work is important for health. In fact, many of us use it as a therapeutic measure for cardiac patients, both in rehabilitation after a heart attack and in keeping them well."

In our own experience, 90 percent of our patients surviving a heart attack go back to previous work and enjoy it.

GOING HOME

After a patient is able to leave the hospital bed, it usually takes an additional week to achieve full ambulation—to be able to walk about readily. Generally, at that point, he is ready to go home.

Once home, he may need another three to six weeks before he is prepared, both physically and psychologically, to return to work.

If you have had a heart attack and have just returned home, your physician will undoubtedly ask you to take things easy at first, to acclimate yourself. He may suggest that you climb no stairs until after a week or so, when you may begin to climb them slowly.

During the period of convalescence, your physician may suggest

that your diet be one limited in calories, free of gas-forming foods
and moderate in salt content.

Again, we stress, obesity must be avoided. If you are overweight,
you should be on a diet. Rid of the need to pump blood to feed
useless fatty tissue, your heart has more energy for more con-
structive activities. And you can count, too, on feeling generally
more fit when you get rid of excess pounds.

Remember, you should not resort to fad diets or any kind of
overly drastic diet. You need your doctor's counseling on how to
go about dieting, and he will be glad to provide it.

If you are not very much overweight and if your dietary habits
have been generally good in the past, your doctor may say that
all you need do is to eat smaller amounts than you have been
accustomed to eat. Or he may advise that you eliminate pastries,
bread, candy, cake, butter, pork and cream, and rely more on
vegetables, lean meats, whole grains and skimmed milk.

If you are considerably overweight, your doctor may do some
figuring about the energy you will be expending and the calories
you will be burning up in the next weeks and months, and tell
you how many fewer calories you can safely consume each day to
bring your weight down in a reasonable period.

CONTROLLING YOUR ARTERY DISEASE

Your heart attack, as you know, came from atherosclerosis. That
atherosclerosis is still present when you recover. Even if a coronary
attack produces such minimal damage to the heart muscle itself
and is responsible for such a sharp increase in collateral circulation that, by and large, the patient is in a healthier position than
before the attack, it is still desirable to do everything possible to
halt or retard the atherosclerotic process.

Research has been finding many factors that appear to be
involved in atherosclerosis. For example, if you have high blood
pressure, it can and will be treated because it is a factor. Elevated
levels of cholesterol and other fats in the blood will be treated
by diet and, if necessary, by medication. A fuller discussion of

these and other factors, and what can be done about them, appears in Chapter 14.

EXERCISE

Lack of sufficient exercise may be an important element in the development of atherosclerosis. While we discuss exercise in Chapter 14 as a means of helping to avoid heart attacks, it deserves discussion here for the patient who has recovered from a heart attack.

Usually, a recovered patient is able to take walks, play golf, fish, swim and engage in many other activities without trouble. Physicians today believe that exercise in moderation is beneficial so long as it causes no pain, shortness of breath or other symptoms.

Some physicians now encourage selected patients to engage in progressively more vigorous exercise once the damaged area of the heart has healed. This is a great change from the days when the emphasis was on sheltering a patient and protecting him from strenuous activity.

Exercise enhances health in many ways. What can it do for the recovered heart-attack patient?

First, if the body can be exercised without pain, the heart will be undergoing conditioning. A heart conditioned to operate at more than just a sedentary level becomes able to operate with greater efficiency, studies show. Both at rest and during activity, a conditioned heart has to beat fewer times per minute. It pumps blood more effectively with each beat. It has longer rest periods between beats. And it requires less oxygen.

Breathing, too, improves with exercise. The lungs take in more air. And oxygen is transported to and taken up by body tissues with greater efficiency.

Exercise also helps to reduce the level of cholesterol and other fatty substances in the blood. And there is evidence from animal studies that exercise stimulates the development of collateral circulation for the heart muscle.

The ideal time for starting an exercise program after recovery from a heart attack has not yet been established, but studies to determine that time are under way. In some experimental programs, very carefully graded exercise is begun while the patient is still in the hospital. In any case, it would seem that most patients should be ready to begin exercise by the end of three months after the attack and preferably before returning to work. Some physicians first test the patient in the office by putting him through some mild standard exercise and then checking his ECG to make certain that no abnormal rhythm develops in response to the activity.

To begin with, exercise may be as simple as walking around the block three times a day when weather permits. The physician may then advise longer walks and then brisker ones, and possibly even brief spurts of jogging.

It is to be expected that after long weeks of inactivity, the pulse will race a bit and there will be some fatigue and breathlessness at first. Gradually, most patients are able to become increasingly active without discomfort.

There have been many studies to measure the effects of progressive exercising on cardiac patients. In one, eighteen men who had heart attacks volunteered to participate in a six-week program. They ranged in age from forty-four to sixty-six, and they were carefully evaluated by electrocardiographic and other tests before the program.

The program consisted of repetitive exercises, including swimming, running and calisthenics, which could be performed an increasing number of times until the patient showed some abnormal response. The patients progressed at individual rates. If an abnormal response appeared, the patient was not allowed to move to a higher level of exercise. If the response was normal, the patient went on to more and more repetitions.

After the six-week period, the patients were again evaluated. The majority of them reported enthusiastically that it was now much easier for them to work out. And more than half demonstrated in the electrocardiographic and other tests measurable evidence of improved heart function.

It seems clear that a carefully adjusted physical-fitness program, carried out with the advice of the physician and with his periodic evaluation of the patient, represents a valuable approach. In addition to helping the patient physically, it helps mentally. Investigators have reported that patients are often relieved of anxiety and depression. Their whole outlook often improves.

GOING BACK TO WORK

As we have said, the vast majority of patients who have had a heart attack can go back to work. Usually, they go back to their old jobs.

Most of them can do almost any kind of work for which they have had the training and experience. There are some, perhaps 10 percent of the total, who may be advised to switch to work which is less demanding physically.

In evaluating an individual patient's capacity, the physician can use exercise tests. He can observe the patient during activity, note the presence or absence of symptoms, and if symptoms develop note their nature and the effort that causes them.

In some cities, heart associations have organized work-evaluation clinics where physicians can send their patients for tests and recommendations about the kinds of physical demands they are capable of meeting.

Many studies reveal that people with heart disease do well on the job. For example, one study by the U.S. Department of Labor compared 1,840 "cardiac" workers with 3,055 workers without heart disease in more than fifty different industries. Measured by productivity, absenteeism and rates of accidents, the workers with heart conditions did as well, and in many cases better, than their fellow workers without heart disease.

Some patients worry that if they go back to work they will be exhausted by the end of the work day. This is not true for the vast majority. Patients who return to work and follow medical advice about diet, exercise, relaxation and other matters do remarkably well. They have energy enough for their work and for leisure-time and social activities.

PAIN

After recovering from a heart attack, not everyone has pain. Some, however, do experience angina with physical overactivity or intense emotion, or after eating a heavy meal. For them, the physician can prescribe nitroglycerin pills, which can quickly end the pain when it occurs and may be used to prevent the pain from developing. Often, over a period of time, as collateral circulation improves, the patient has less and less trouble with angina.

SEXUAL LIFE

Are marital relations harmful after convalescence? This question often worries patients, and it is wise for them to discuss it with their physicians. Usually the answer is no, they are not harmful.

Generally, if there are no complications during recovery, a patient may be advised to return to sexual activity by about the sixth week after leaving the hospital. We often suggest that at least at first the spouse undertake most of the activity and that the patient remain as passive as possible during the sex act.

Intercourse does increase blood pressure, pulse rate and the work of the heart, but by the time they are six weeks out of the hospital—and thus usually about ten weeks past their heart attack—most patients do well. Very few have angina during intercourse. If they do, the physician may instruct them to take a nitroglycerin pill just before.

We still encounter some patients who are fearful of resuming marital relations. They have the idea that many heart attacks occur during intercourse. This is not the case at all. We sometimes urge tense and anxious male patients to go away with their wives, even if for no more than a weekend; to go off someplace, any place, where they can relax; and to resume sexual relations in the relaxed atmosphere.

SOCIAL LIFE

A heart attack need not, and certainly should not, make you a social invalid any more than it should make you a physical invalid. Can you resume your former social life, hobbies and other activities? Chances are that you can, though if they were excessive in the past your physician may advise some moderation.

You will be guided, too, by your own reactions. If, in the beginning, you feel fatigued after work, it makes sense to go to bed early. As you become accustomed to the work routine again, the fatigue is likely to diminish and finally disappear. If you tolerate a day's work and an evening of social activity, there is no reason why you should not enjoy doing so. Any time that you can spend with cheerful, optimistic friends is time well spent; cheer and optimism are what anyone recovering from an illness needs.

CLIMATE

Some patients ask about moving to a Southern climate after a heart attack. Making a permanent move, uprooting oneself and one's family, leaving behind job, friends and other ties is not easy. Nor is it usually essential. The upset from such a move may exact more of a toll than does cold and blustery weather.

It is a fact that walking against a cold winter wind and plodding through snow increase the work of the heart. If a patient has had a very severe heart attack, he may do better in a warm Southern climate—and so, if it is possible, we advise him to take a midwinter vacation in such a climate.

In hot weather, air conditioning is a comfort for anyone and particularly for a heart patient. Very high temperatures add to the work of the heart. Air conditioning can reduce the work load and may be most helpful in curbing any anginal attacks.

DRIVING

Driving is a matter of some importance for the heart patient. Tests show that driving can put the circulatory system under stress even in young, healthy people. A study carried out in England revealed that just getting into a car causes an increase in heart rate, perhaps in anticipation of the task ahead.

In an investigation carried out with 600 healthy drivers, 80 percent were found to experience a 10 percent increase in pulse rate while driving on a lightly traveled road, while in city traffic their pulse rate increased by more than 20 percent. In addition, blood pressure rose by nearly one-third in 11 percent of the subjects when they drove on rural roads and in 28 percent while they drove in urban traffic.

More studies are needed before any firm guidelines can be established regarding driving practices of cardiac patients.

Meanwhile, it may be advisable for patients in the first few months after recovery from a heart attack not to drive and subject the heart to the extra burden. Later, they may begin to drive in leisurely fashion and for short trips. Thereafter, the driving may be increased.

It is important to point out here that a patient's driving temperament must be considered. If driving makes him unduly tense, if he becomes easily aggravated by other drivers and by traffic conditions, the stress on his heart may be considerable and he would probably do best to leave the car at home.

SMOKING

Smoking is a health hazard for anyone. In addition to its association with lung cancer, cigarette smoking has been linked with heart disease. We discuss this in more detail in Chapter 14.

There is less risk from cigar or pipe smoking, possibly because cigar and pipe smokers do not usually inhale.

Certainly, for the person who has had a heart attack, any

factor which may be involved in coronary atherosclerosis is to be avoided if at all possible. We urge our patients to stop smoking cigarettes or, at the very least, to reduce their smoking.

ALCOHOL

Alcohol has a relaxing effect and in moderate quantities may be helpful for some patients. We permit many patients to have 3 to 4 ounces daily, especially during a relaxing cocktail hour before dinner.

But please note: Alcohol in excess can be harmful for anyone and for the cardiac patient in particular. It can lead to undesirable weight gain. In addition, alcohol in excess stresses the heart muscle and may provoke angina and even congestive heart failure. If alcohol is used, it should be in moderation.

COFFEE AND TEA

Once coffee and tea were strictly proscribed. Both are stimulants and it was therefore supposed that their effects would be bad: that they would increase heart action and perhaps produce abnormal rhythms.

We know now that these beverages have vasodilating effects, too—and such opening up of arteries may help a little in nourishing the heart muscle. But moderation is the key. If you are a heavy coffee or tea drinker, your physician may advise that you limit yourself to one or two cups a day.

TALK OUT YOUR FEELINGS

Every patient experiences anxiety after a heart attack. All his life he has thought of heart disease in terms of sudden death. He may conclude all too readily that his heart will totally fail to function sometime in the near future. He may express his anxiety or leave it unspoken.

We stress again that it is important to express it, to talk it over with a physician, to understand that there is no shame in feeling it, that it is common, and that it is healthy to discuss your fears. The very act of discussing them is helpful. For bottled-up anxiety produces tension, and you are better off simply from the act of removing the cork.

But, beyond that, the physician can help. He can provide not glib, general reassurance, but answers to your questions, information you can chew on. He can provide new and additional understanding for you about what happened during your heart attack, what has been happening since, what has been done about it, what your condition is now, what your capabilities are, and what will happen in the future.

There are several types of psychological reactions patients may go through after a heart attack.

One is an obvious type of excessive anxiety. The patient is unduly anxious about his heart. His whole state of mind is apprehensive. His facial expression is anxious. He has difficulty sleeping.

A second type of reaction amounts to an excessive defense against anxiety. The abnormal anxiety is there but buried, and the patient shows only, and may only be conscious of, the measures he is using to keep his anxiety buried. He may make great efforts to stay calm at all times, to avoid fast walking or any seemingly undue exertion, to control his diet, and to follow doctor's orders so meticulously that he is sure to take every pill on time to the second.

When either of these reactions is present, the physician can help by showing the patient that it is an abnormal complication. He can help the patient to understand that it has developed because of nagging doubts and unanswered questions. He can encourage the patient to talk about the doubts and ask the questions, and he can answer the questions and resolve many and possibly all of the doubts.

A third type of reaction is the complete denial of anxiety. The patient acts as though he has not had a heart attack. He may rush around, engage in the most vigorous of sports and in other strenuous activities, daring to do what men without heart disease would not do. And he is not pretending; rather, he is using a psychological mechanism which denies the existence of any facts that would produce anxiety. The physician can help such a patient by showing him what he is doing, what the mechanism is, and what the potential dangers are.

Depression is another type of reaction. It is perfectly normal after a heart attack for a person to go through a period of days and even weeks or months during which he feels blue. Until the heart attack, if he gave any thought to his health it may have been to consider that he was totally healthy. Suddenly, that idea has been snatched away. He sees himself at first as most unhealthy, as a total invalid. But, as his physical recovery progresses, he loses that idea. He is not an invalid. He begins to regain confidence that he can win back health. And as this happens his depression goes.

Such depression is normal. But in a few patients, severe and extended depression develops. Their blues are overwhelming. They have feelings of worthlessness and guilt. They become withdrawn, apathetic. For such patients, too, the physician can do much by resolving doubts and answering questions and, when necessary, by using antidepressant drugs.

REPEAT ATTACKS

If you've had a heart attack, must there be another? No.

No one can be certain whether a person will have a repeat attack. But it is definitely a fact that a second attack is not inevitable. Nor, incidentally, is it true that a second attack, if it occurs, is more serious than the first; and that if a third attack occurs, it is inevitably fatal. Patients have had very minor second and third attacks. Many patients have recovered from four, five and six attacks.

Your best chance of living comfortably without further attacks will lie in heeding your doctor's recommendations about your weight, your diet, your work, your exercise and your rest and relaxation. And a thoughtful reading of Chapter 14 on preventive measures will be helpful to you. While your heart attack has clearly shown that you have atherosclerosis, the use of current knowledge about factors associated with the development of atherosclerosis can be valuable in helping to prevent it from getting worse.

You may actually make headway against the problem. If, as your collateral circulation develops, you can slow down or stop further development of atherosclerosis, you will achieve a net gain on the side of improved circulation for your heart.

Remember, the outlook for coronary patients is better now than it has ever been before, better even than just a few years ago, and with all the research now under way it is certain to become better still.

[12]

A Personal Experience:
A Physician Has a
Heart Attack

Even after more than fifteen years, the details and the impact remain clear.

My health had always been remarkably good. Indeed, I took for granted my ability to endure all forms of physical or mental stress without penalty—particularly those so well known to practicing physicians: irregular and inadequate sleep, sporadic exercise, unreasonable working hours and emotional strain.

It is not difficult to explain how one becomes a person accustomed to a full burden of activity and anxiety. A combination of ego-motivation and disciplined training is an essential ingredient. In my younger days, this was flavored with the belief that the practice of medicine implied full devotion to others and none to self. Additionally, the Great Depression left the conviction that one had to keep moving if one expected to eat.

Regardless of how it all came about, I was engaged in a running contest between increasing obligations and the energy to honor them. Each day brought a critical deadline. Furthermore, I was part of a new, exciting but trying effort of medicine—a team effort in heart surgery—involving close cooperation between medical cardiologists, surgical cardiologists, anesthetists, cardiac physiologists and others. I functioned as one of the medical cardiologists on the team, which was headed by the most enterprising, aggressive and innovative of the world's heart surgeons. My duties included selecting patients for surgical treatment, developing better techniques for selection and evaluating the results of operations and the reasons for success and failure. These functions were performed at Hahnemann Medical College and Hospital in Philadelphia, but were combined with lecture and teaching tours throughout the country. In brief, I was working at one of the frontiers of medicine and was deeply concerned about pushing back the frontier.

The moments I spent away from work were as crowded as the work day itself: golf, tennis, swimming, social engagements.

EARLY WARNING

It is difficult to explain how an active physician can remain completely ignorant of his own physical health. In my case, there was a wide divergence between my actual physical state and my estimation of that state, and this persisted even in the face of some adequate warnings.

I recall undergoing an insurance examination several months prior to the heart attack. The insurance examiner arrived when I was making rounds on the sixteenth floor of the hospital. I had forgotten the appointment, and when my default became apparent and I was interrupted in my work, I impatiently raced down the fire stairs rather than waiting for the elevator and dashed across the street to my office, where the insurance doctor was. He began to make the usual observations and recordings after a decent interval in which he was waiting for me to catch my breath. After repeated attempts to obtain an acceptable blood pressure and pulse rate, he abandoned the project.

"You're apparently in miserable physical condition or are actually ill," he said. "In any event, I can't approve your application at the present time. I will repeat the examination a few days later." He was an old hand at the job, had a dour personality, hardly apologized for his decision and emphasized its finality by leaving me standing there.

Regrettably, I viewed his remarks as the drivel that might be expected from a physician who knew precious little about his profession. I was more annoyed by the inconvenience of another examination than curious about the reasons that made it necessary. Ten days later I was reexamined when I was more at ease, and a normal blood pressure and pulse were recorded. I forgot the incident and its ominous implications.

In retrospect, the denial of vulnerability which this and a score of other instances illustrate appears almost pathological. My father had had coronary heart disease at a relatively young age; my older brother also suffered from the ailment. I could hardly claim ignorance about the basic problem or about the likelihood that I was particularly vulnerable.

But we deny our mortality, and thus feel no concern about the possibility of health failure. A child's fantasy often revolves about the belief that he will live forever. The front-line soldier often is convinced that a lethal bullet may strike anyone but him. In the same way, the healthy, hard-working human may deny his vulnerability to body ache or destruction.

A SLOWLY EVOLVING HEART ATTACK

The weekend of my attack was a particularly hot and humid one. I had promised to join some neighbors in a tennis match. Spring had been tardy. I had had little exercise over the winter and was not prepared for vigorous exercise. If that reflects an unhealthy pattern of living, the fact that I nevertheless proceeded to play reflects how accustomed I had become to taking my health for granted.

Each of the three neighbors who joined me for that match was over forty and equally guilty of lack of preparedness. I imagine their work loads were slightly less than that of a physician, but at least two of them were considerably stouter than I and smoked cigarettes with equal or greater frequency.

It is not to be presumed, because all of us involved in the

tennis match were over forty and out of condition, that we were of small athletic ability. On the contrary, two of us had played on college teams, and one easily could have. Each was motivated to win through habit and personality. The playing was vigorous.

We were at midmatch when, after a hard run across court and a futile effort to retrieve a beautifully angled shot, I felt a peculiar sensation in my midchest.

As we have said, the pain of a heart attack can be sudden, unrelenting, and the cause of an onrush of fear—or so mild that it is mistaken for indigestion and causes just a vague uneasiness. I was quite familiar with its symptoms. Indeed, on thousands of occasions I had applied my knowledge to other humans with reasonable accuracy and assurance. And yet, in my own case I was not quick to recognize that the uneasy feeling I had in my chest was in truth a major cardiac catastrophe.

I did feel uneasy. I did pause and look around as if to see whether anyone else had noticed my uneasiness. I rubbed my chest. The discomfort persisted; it grew in intensity; and even as I turned to walk back to my station on the court I knew I could not continue to play. It wasn't that the pain was so intense or that fear overwhelmed me. I just knew it would be impossible for me to continue to run and play.

As if to seal the decision, the racket fell from my hand. I picked it up and excused myself briefly with a superficial explanation that I was simply too tired to go on. I walked slowly back home. By the time I got there, the pain had largely subsided. I showered, rested briefly, then dressed to greet guests who had just arrived.

I spent an uneasy night, but my discomfort lacked character. Perhaps the most significant feeling was utter fatigue. The following day I returned to work, had the usual type of day, and that evening, with a number of colleagues, celebrated in proper banquet style an approaching marriage. At the conclusion of the meal I began to feel the uneasiness in my chest again but the discomfort was mild. On my return home, I went promptly to bed and did so without any worry that a disaster was about to mature.

This story I recite of a slowly evolving heart attack is not unusual. Many attacks mature over a period of twenty-four to seventy-two hours. During this interval, repeated bouts of discomfort occur but subside, either spontaneously or in response to a nonspecific form of medication such as a digestant or sedative. It is not an easy matter to obtain a clear history of the slow evolution of a heart attack, for in many instances the early pains are so insignificant that they are forgotten by the patient. Almost invariably, however, the patient will confess that for a period of time prior to the actual heart attack the sensation of fatigue was very marked. Every clinician of any experience has learned that fatigability is a premonitory sign of coronary occlusion.

I had been guilty of a grave error in not seeking medical care at the very outset of my discomfort. About half the patients with heart attacks do not reach medical facilities alive. The best hope, obviously, of getting medical help in time is to report symptoms as soon as they develop. As a physician, I knew quite well what was the most likely cause of the discomforts I felt. My failure to report these symptoms immediately to a physician was inexcusable.

The final attack of pain felt as if someone had struck me in the solar plexus. The pain radiated into my left shoulder and upper arm. I had almost fallen asleep when it came. I had to sit upright without knowing why and almost immediately thereafter to stand at the bedside. The upright position was comforting but the pain persisted. Suddenly, accompanying it, was a sensation of tumultuous irregular beating in the chest. At first there was just a hesitant skip or two, then a twitter and finally a giant pounding with shorter and longer pauses.

The physician who came was a classmate and friend. He had earned his stripes in general practice before concentrating in the specialty of otolaryngology. He recognized the likelihood that my discomfort was cardiac in origin. He gave me an injection and when, within an hour, the pain had subsided and I began to drift into drug-induced stupor, he left, having accomplished what he could. Plans were to be made at a more reasonable hour for additional care depending on the clinical picture.

I remained quiet for a short period of time. I was awakened

not so much by pain as by the tumultuous beating in my chest. My thoughts fought for expression through a very thick haze of Demerol. Despite the drug, I deduced that ventricular tachy-cardia—abnormally rapid beating of the ventricles—was present in short bursts, and I spent the remainder of that wicked night administering quinidine sulfate to myself. As I did so, my heart rhythm became more normal, permitting me some sleep.

What was happening at the time of my coronary is very simple to explain in terms of current knowledge. I was having electrical failure. The damage to the heart muscle had set up electrical-conduction disturbances and a potentially lethal rhythm—a rhythm which could wear out the heart in a short period of time or turn into ventricular fibrillation, an ineffective twitching of the heart muscle, and progress to cardiac arrest, complete heart standstill.

Ventricular tachycardia today is recognized as a major problem to be treated in a hospital coronary care or intensive-care unit. Prompt recognition and treatment have saved many lives.

Although the critical nature of this rhythm was known at the time I became ill, methods of treatment were not so clearly defined as now and there were no special facilities in hospitals. So what I am describing is a bold but foolish approach to the problem. My attempt to correct the arrhythmia by administering quinidine at home might be considered, in view of the lack of special facilities at that time, not so grave a default as it would be now. But self-treatment at any time is a basically inexcusable venture.

The next morning I was seen by my immediate superior at the medical school, who came to the house with an electrocardiograph. The tracing indicated clearly that I had had a coronary occlusion with myocardial infarction, death of some muscle tissue in the front part of the heart. The damage was extensive.

My superior's approach to the problem was to insist on hospi-talization at once. My reaction was immediate and loud: I re-fused to go. It is difficult to explain my motivation. I suppose part of the reason was that I did not want to underscore my weakness—if illness is a weakness—by being bedded down in a public institution. Also, of course, in times of distress, the comforts of home beckon.

The battle was quickly and properly lost.

HOSPITALIZATION

In reflecting on those first days in the hospital, I cannot help but note how much more sophisticated treatment is today than it was when I had my heart attack. At that time, cardiac monitors for detecting abnormal rhythms were unknown. The nature of my heart rhythm was determined sporadically during the day by a nurse or physician. In between these checks, however, potentially lethal rhythms could have occurred and recurred scores of times without being noted and treated. The medications were limited, too. And there were no refined methods of assessing the working capacity of the heart such as exist now. The heart could have failed, and early warnings of the disaster would not have been observed; even if they were, there was then only a single drug that might help, in contrast to the many now available.

As we have noted, the early days after a severe heart attack can be uncertain ones because of possible complications. Apparently, I was threatened by none. Slowly but steadily I progressed to a convalescent state.

The time for full realization eventually came. At first drugs had dulled the senses. Then denial entered the picture, taking the form of lethargy, sleep, reluctance to think thoroughly about what had happened. But the realization that a major health accident had occurred finally did come and with it a profound depression.

I do not have the benefit of psychiatric training, but some facts about the psyche have become evident to me over the years. I suppose, as I said, that the most significant insult to the ego is the emotional and intellectual acknowledgment of vulnerability to death—an acknowledgment that plays havoc with the fantasy of immortality.

Depression often includes self-pity. In the depths of emotional despair, a patient can drift away from loved ones, even holding them in part responsible for his fate, and can turn on friends and regret that it was not they who were afflicted. Finally, he can withdraw into himself and remain uncommunicative.

Depression is not unusual and in a sense not abnormal. How long it persists and the emotional state which succeeds it, however, are critical. If the depression is followed by a sense of well-being almost to the point of euphoria, then the patient is denying the original accident and remains in psychic imbalance. If the depression continues unabated, again the patient's psychic balance has been impaired. But if the depression is succeeded by a frank realization that an important health disturbance has occurred, and if the patient therefore prepares himself emotionally to make the proper adjustments, he is returning to normal.

My depression was significant and prolonged. It started as an indifference to events about me. They held no interest for me if I couldn't be part of them. When I had been well and all too busy, I had cherished the thought of moments of relaxation when I might reflect, read or write without being beset by daily events. Now that I was on the way to recovery, could sit up without difficulty and had the opportunity to catch up with the mountain of material that needed to be read, digested and written, I was disinterested. I drifted into an intellectual stupor. The depression was almost a pleasant sensation. It was a complete withdrawal—to a safe, comfortable place in which I was determined to stay.

I am not certain whether recovery occurred spontaneously or was the result of persistent encouragement by nurses and physicians. Father A may well have been involved.

I am not a religious man, nor am I a Catholic. Nevertheless, Father A possessed a combination of congeniality, kindliness, compassion and fervor that I found soothing. He was an old friend. Assigned to the hospital and specifically to the area of heart surgery, he would visit patients daily, and in addition to offering them comfort he provided some for the physicians who were trying to mature heart surgery into a helpful form of therapy.

It was natural for Father A to visit with me during my illness. It was the man, not the blessings he pronounced—it was the way he spent the time with me, weaving together what was going on in my room with what was happening outside—that made the large difference to me.

Another touching, compassionate event influenced me in this period of depression. I had trained at Peter Bent Brigham Hospital in Boston under Dr. Samuel Levine. He was recognized as one of the foremost minds in cardiology. I developed a strong affection for him. Apparently he returned that affection and held to the hope that I might one day score a point or two in the field in which he excelled. Indeed, it was he who had encouraged me in the early days of cardiac surgery to persist in my efforts in this area.

At the time of my attack, he too was hospitalized—for a serious surgical procedure. When he heard that I was ill, he requested his physicians' permission to go to Philadelphia at the earliest possible moment to assist in my care. He was refused permission because he was barely on the road to recovery. He listened respectfully and that same evening got dressed, walked out of the hospital, drove to the airport, and came to Philadelphia. Later, he returned to Boston and the hospital, apparently none the worse for his experience.

I date my first real feeling of confidence from the moment Dr. Levine walked into my room, questioned me about the nature of my attack, examined me and assured me of my recovery. Professionally, I realized that his reasons for assurance were no more securely based than anyone else's, but the way he spoke, the conviction with which he made his comments, provided great comfort.

As I gradually recovered from the depression, I began to read. I read voraciously. I began to think, too, about a return to professional activity. Now each little event became significant to me: the moment when I first dangled my feet out of bed; the time I was first permitted to use the bathroom; the time I first shaved myself.

CONVALESCENCE

I came home at the end of six weeks. It had been an inter-
minably long period: four of the weeks spent in absolute bed
rest, two in gradual rehabilitation. As we have seen, the custom
is different today: sometimes, if a patient's condition has sta-
bilized, he will be out of bed within seventy-two to ninety-six
hours after a heart attack.

When the patient can be permitted out of bed earlier—and,
obviously, not all can—rehabilitation can be accomplished more
readily. There is less of the weakening of muscles that occurs
with prolonged bed rest; there is healthier blood flow.

At the time of my hospitalization, however, the concept of
early ambulation was in its infancy. It wasn't used in my case.
As a result it took me almost two weeks to learn how to walk
again.

The trip home was made by ambulance without incident. I
entered my house on a stretcher and immediately was greeted
by my dog Brownie, who leaped on the stretcher and rode the
stairs with me.

But the warmth and comfort of home, the return to familiar
scenes, led to another period of depression. I think this was
brought on by the realization that I still had considerable physical
disability. For example, I could not walk down the hallway from
my bedroom to the end of the house without hesitancy. As I took
my weak, wavering steps, I could not help but think of how
many times I had run up and down this hallway with ease. I
looked longingly down the steps to the first floor. Restrictions
prevented me from trying more than a few of them at a time.
I remembered when I had bounded up those steps.

As I remembered more and more the things I could once do, I
felt increasingly useless and a burden for everybody about me.
This depression, if anything, was more severe than the one in
the hospital. It took the form now of outrageous impatience with
everyone about me, including my wife and children. I held them
responsible for my slow progress, for one ridiculous reason or

another. I resented their involvement with the world and my exclusion from it. I interpreted their instructions to me, all of which were restrictive, as indicating their further interest in keeping me from the world. My depression was now laced with anxiety and perhaps some paranoia.

One of the young men whom I had trained in medicine during my own medical residency had become a psychiatrist. He was an early visitor and after the first visit returned at unusually frequent intervals. He had noticed my disturbance and set about in a quiet, intelligent way to try to correct it by coming several times a week to speak with me and hear me out. I am certain his visits were helpful even though there was no obvious attempt to engage in psychotherapy.

I had been an inveterate smoker. With my coronary, I had stopped. But when I returned home, I found that I had not been emancipated from the habit as I had believed. The desire to smoke was particularly acute after meals. Nevertheless, I resisted it.

The relationship between smoking and heart disease was less well known then than it is now. That was the period when it was first being realized that there was a statistical relationship between smoking and lung cancer; and evidence connecting heart disease and smoking was less impressive. Yet the easiest figure to remember now is one that was worked out very early: a person who smokes after having a heart attack will, on the average, live three years less than the individual who gives up smoking. I was impressed by that; I felt that an added three years might allow me to see a child through college or to honor some other equally important obligation.

My intake of fat had been restricted in the hospital; I continued to restrict fats when I returned home.

Our home is a comfortable one, located in a beautiful area of Philadelphia, with ample open space for walking. Following instructions, I gradually undertook walking, starting with the equivalent of a city block and extending this block by block until I was walking a mile twice a day. My dog's companionship was helpful. Strength in my limbs returned slowly.

Fear was present and took various forms: hesitation to cross a street for fear I might be caught in traffic; hesitation about walking up a slight incline for fear it might precipitate disaster; fear that some vague discomfort in the general area of the chest (actually of no cardiac significance) might represent a new attack. Perhaps it seems strange that a physician trained in the field could not differentiate the meaningful from the meaningless; it may have been that I knew, as the popular saying goes, too much.

After almost six weeks at home, though, I felt much better physically and mentally, reassured because there had been no recurrence of pain and no delayed complication.

THE RETURN TO WORK

It had been three months since the heart attack, and I was to be permitted to resume the practice of medicine. But my instructions were precise: At the outset, two to three hours a day, no more. And, at least in the beginning, no night calls. I had made many night calls before, not house calls but calls in response to critical situations in the hospital. My particular interest in cardiac surgery made these night calls necessary very frequently. But this obligation was to be turned over to several associates for the time being.

The practice of medicine on a part-time basis is not easy. Patients learn to consider their doctors as firm barriers between themselves and illness. The fact that a physician himself is ill shakes their confidence, makes them feel insecure. Moreover, the fact that a physician has the very disease in which he is presumably an expert casts doubt both on his ability and his understanding of the problem. Actually, however, the physician who has been through the various phases of an illness has a better understanding of and may have greater empathy for his patients.

I expected to lose some patients, and yet I was disappointed when I did. I was upset by something else: the finding that even now I became very easily fatigued. Perhaps of all the difficulties which may remain after an acute coronary, the most disturbing—next to angina—is the lack of ability to make a physical effort without becoming tired.

Some patients have angina pectoris after recovering from a heart attack. It may occur because certain areas of the heart muscle are still not receiving adequate blood flow. I had no residual angina—but, as I said, I was disturbed by the fatigue.

Fatigue is a curious complaint in cardiacs. It appears to result from the fact that the body may somewhat reduce the blood flow to muscles in the arms, legs and elsewhere during activity in order to maintain as large as possible a flow to more critical areas such as the brain and lungs. It is as if the body instinctively puts the blood where it can do the most good.

When flow to the muscles is reduced, the muscles not only lack adequate nourishment but have built up in them waste substances that are not adequately washed away by the smaller amount of blood. These waste substances irritate nerve fibers in the muscle and give rise to the symptom of fatigue.

I returned to work tired, and that was discomforting. I was disturbed, too, that the return to work did not immediately eliminate completely my depressed feelings and bouts of moodiness. I suppose I was also psychologically disturbed to find that the world had continued without interruption despite my serious illness and that my patients had received care and had developed new relationships. In short, my ego was rather deeply dashed by the realization that life goes on quite successfully regardless of any one individual's misfortune.

I recite these small details because I suspect that the same reactions occur in most patients afflicted with serious heart disease. I think they occur in people with other forms of illness, too, but perhaps not quite so acutely.

Actually, I had not been back at work for very long before I began to realize that a number of patients were booking appointments to come to talk to me to see how a physician reacted to the problem they themselves had. They wanted to know, for example, the nature and location of my pain; how I had withstood it; how I felt now; what I intended to do about it.

I answered their questions with real empathy. When a patient spoke to me about his fear of death, I could understand him, since I had undergone the very same anxiety. When a patient said that he went to bed at night trembling for fear he might close his eyes and never open them again, I could understand. When patients said that they often walked the floor at night rather than take the chance of falling asleep, I didn't think of them as simply highly neurotic; I had been in their anxious state.

When a patient expressed feelings of guilt for imposing a burden on a spouse, I could appreciate those feelings, too. I could understand very well impotence in a man with heart disease because of fear of death during intercourse—and frigidity in a wife fearful that her ill husband might die during the sex act.

Certainly I had had knowledge of all of this before my illness and had helped patients with these problems. But now I had an even better understanding and a much greater sensitivity.

A PREVENTIVE ROUTINE

The time came when I had to approach my own long-term treatment.

Like everyone else, by the age of forty I had rather fixed dietary habits. I was not eager to make changes. Yet I approached the problem as rationally as I could and did put myself on a low-fat diet because it was a reasonable concept and the restrictions were not unbearable.

The benefits of exercise cannot be obtained unless there is regular, reasoned activity. This had not been my exercise pattern in the past; I had been active sporadically and not wisely, sometimes going to extremes after weeks of virtually no activity at all.

Now I was required to develop an exercise routine that I could follow regularly. I determined that I would use walking as my major exercise and, as I said, began soon after returning home from the hospital. I kept up my walks and enjoyed them—and, later, found myself again enjoying other activities, such as leisurely swimming and dancing.

I gave up smoking, though not, as I have indicated, without difficulty. I had tried to stop on many occasions before on the general theory that smoking could impair health. It can be difficult, however, to break the smoking habit on the basis of general theory alone. Motivation has to be great for many of us belonging to the so-called "hooked generation." But motivation was high for me now. I was fearful of the disease I had, and I was not about to help it destroy me.

I worked from late September until December, gradually increasing my work hours. Twice a week I left the office at three in the afternoon and went to a health center, where I had a massage and nap before returning home. On other afternoons, I left the office around four and rested before dinner. I sought less strenuous forms of entertainment. Instead of the physicians' parties to which we had been committed, my wife and I purchased a box for the Philadelphia Orchestra's Saturday-night concerts and thoroughly enjoyed a pleasure we had denied ourselves before.

And so a new pace was established. It was not unpleasant. Indeed, the new life had distinct advantages over the old. Both my wife and I felt that we were now more the masters of our fate than before. People no longer expected impossible tasks of us at impossible hours.

It was about this time that a science reporter from one of Philadelphia's daily newspapers approached me about writing an article, "A Physician Has a Heart Attack." The purpose was to tell the background of a heart attack and how it is possible for even a physician to find himself engulfed by such a catastrophe. I gave the reporter the facts and told him of my training program and my hopes and expectations for the future, emphasizing that people do recover and return to productive living.

The article attracted interest. Apparently, the public had been convinced that this sort of thing did not happen to physicians, although statistics indicate clearly that physicians are among the most vulnerable. At any rate, shortly after the article appeared I became identified as the cardiologist with the heart attack, even though I am certain there were scores of others in this area in the same situation.

My battle with depression was not completely finished, though I don't think it evolved from some previous subtle psychic imbalance. I had not been a moody person prior to the heart attack,

had not been given to extremes of temper. I had not been trained
in Freudian principles and I did not "play around" with them.
Simply, I had become depressed because of an acute health
insult.

Early in December I felt it necessary to break off from work.
Mild depression was partly responsible for the decision. But, in
the main, I was attempting to develop a pattern of taking periodic
vacations and thought that the vacation season around Christmas
was a good one.

Several years before my coronary, a patient had come from San
Juan, Puerto Rico, for cardiac surgery and had been placed under
my care. She was a delightful woman who had arrived with her
husband, daughter and grandchild. In keeping with Old World
custom, all members of the family had insisted on trying to
register at the hospital, maintaining that the family even in
illness could not be separated. We made special arrangements
to accommodate the patient's daughter and convinced the others
they would do best to stay at a hotel.

The patient was admitted to the hospital with a diagnosis
of mitral-valve defect from rheumatic heart disease. But the
true diagnosis was atrial septal defect, an opening in the septum
between the right and left atrial chambers. She was operated on
successfully, though hers was an unusually difficult operation at
that stage in the development of cardiac surgery. She recovered
and departed for San Juan, grateful for the kindness, attention
and care she had received.

When she learned of my heart attack, she called from San
Juan, asking that I come to convalesce there. The family owned
a large private island—Palaminos in the Caribbean—where I
could be free of all obligations and just bask in the sun.

In December, my wife and two daughters accompanied me
to Puerto Rico. We spent the next four weeks in the area, dividing
our time between the island of Palaminos and the yacht which
our friends owned.

I mark this vacation well because I think it was really the
beginning of true recovery. All the ingredients were right: concerned friends, devoted family, benign climate, complete relaxa-

tion and opportunity to think myself back to the world at large.

I returned to practice, and soon it was full-time practice. Within a year after the attack, I had begun to lose vivid memory of the life that had been before. The present seemed to have been forever. And it was a good present. So it remains now, more than fifteen years later.

A heart attack can open the door to a score of complex problems, but it can offer rewards, too. An important one, I think, for many is a new appreciation of life, a new appreciation of the meaningful things in life and how to enjoy them—and perhaps the first opportunity we have allowed ourselves to enjoy them. In my own case, as a physician, I believe very earnestly that I am a better physician for having had an attack, although I would not recommend one as a method of becoming a more able doctor. Nevertheless, I have found that my services to patients are more valuable, and more valued, because I have been through the ordeal.

Finally, I have learned that the preventive routine which I follow—and which I recommend to my patients—is a feasible one. It cannot be presented as an absolute—as a certain means of avoiding all trouble. But it is sensible and practical, and gives rise to a feeling that you are making a contribution to your future well-being.

[13]

The Need for Action

Today more and more Americans, particularly middle-aged men, show concern about heart trouble. They jog and bicycle to bring their weight down; they trim fat off their steaks and spread corn-oil margarine on their toast; many give up cigarettes.

Yet, when a heart attack strikes, they are slow to seek help.

It happens many times every day. The victim may be experiencing all the classic symptoms of a coronary: the chest pain, the cold sweat, the shortness of breath. He knows something is very wrong. And yet he does not call for help. He tries to pass off the symptoms as of no great consequence, to find some other explanation for them—any explanation but heart attack. Not long afterward, within hours, he is dead—not because death was inevitable, but because he didn't act to prevent it.

Each year, more than 1.5 million Americans suffer coronary attacks. Of these, about 600,000 die. And of the 600,000 who die, 400,000 never reach a hospital alive. A large number of the 400,000—perhaps even 150,000 or more—might be saved if there were the chance to treat them, to monitor them closely, to take

162

immediate action to overcome and even prevent the events after a heart attack that lead to sudden death.

In one study covering 160 heart-attack victims treated at two hospitals, the delay between onset of symptoms and hospitalization was found to average three and one-half hours and ranged all the way up to four and five days. Transportation time from home to hospital accounted for only a minute fraction of the delay—an average of just twenty minutes.

Perhaps procrastination is a bit more understandable among patients whose symptoms, though disturbing, are not entirely clear-cut: symptoms of seeming indigestion, with some dizziness and shortness of breath. But 80 percent of the patients in the study had suffered intense chest pain and had nevertheless delayed in calling a doctor.

Other studies have shown that patients often have warning signals—increasingly sharp and frequent episodes of chest pain— as long as a week before the onset of a heart attack and yet disregard them. At one hospital, 65 percent of heart-attack patients had had such warnings.

Often patients excuse their delay on the grounds that they didn't want to bother a physician at night or on a weekend or that they thought the trouble would "go away."

What is the real reason for procrastination?

Unquestionably, in some cases, there may be a failure to understand the significance of symptoms—to realize, for example, that seeming indigestion may herald a heart attack. But more often certain attitudes about heart disease keep people from seeking medical care when they suspect they have heart-disease symptoms. At a recent special conference on the problem held by the American College of Cardiology, the consensus was that people often deny they have symptoms of a heart attack because "they believe it is a completely incapacitating condition from which they will never truly recover."

A similar denial mechanism based on defeatism is responsible for the failure of some people with angina pectoris to seek help before they go on to have heart attacks. Dr. Paul Dudley White has written: "A few of my patients have concealed their angina

pectoris from their families, their friends, and even their physicians until forced by circumstances, for example, an attack of
coronary thrombosis, to admit it. Some of the garment workers
in New York City, upon the discovery of tell-tale evidence in their
electrocardiograms, have confessed having had characteristic chest
pains during the year, which they did not report except as a
transient illness that kept them at home for only a day or two."

HOW ACTION HELPS

More than 80 percent of sudden deaths occur within twenty-
four hours after a heart attack. You might expect that there would
be extensive damage to the heart to account for deaths. But in
many victims of fatal coronaries, the heart muscle is only mini-
mally damaged.

For sudden death after a heart attack can often be compared
to the way a clock will sometimes stop ticking even though its
internal mechanism is still in good working order. What accounts
for the sudden stopping of a heart which is really still basically
sound, still too good to die?

Electrical failure.

After a heart attack and the death of even a small portion of
the heart muscle, the electrical patterns of the heart may be
disturbed. Then, currents from the heart's pacemaker that
initiate heart-muscle contraction and control rhythm will deviate
from normal. With the abnormal surges of current, the heart
rhythm will become abnormal. The heart may go into ventricular
fibrillation—its contractions uneven, uncoordinated. It becomes
a quivering instead of contracting mass and soon the heart stands
still. In effect, the heart has electrocuted itself.

What can be done to prevent this?

At the turn of the century, Swiss physiologists found that they
could change ventricular fibrillation in the heart of dogs back
to normal rhythm by applying strong electric currents to the
heart through the opened chest—currents to shock the heart
back to normal beat.

Thirty years later, William B. Kouwenhoven, a professor of electrical engineering at Johns Hopkins University, developed a practical instrument for delivering current to a fibrillating human heart. Some years afterward, Dr. Paul M. Zoll of Harvard Medical School found that the chest did not have to be opened; an electric shock could be just as effective when delivered through the intact chest wall. Then, in 1960, Dr. Bernard Lown and his colleagues at Harvard Medical School developed a method for delivering a single electric pulse from a capacitor which was even more effective than the alternating current previously used.

Still, resuscitating victims of ventricular fibrillation was only occasionally successful. Rarely was there enough time to get the equipment to the patient. When fibrillation begins, blood circulation virtually ceases; the heart is no longer pumping, only quivering. Within three minutes, serious brain damage develops from the lack of blood. And, for lack of blood to the heart muscle, damage there is also increased and may become so great that within a few minutes after fibrillation begins the heart can no longer be returned to normal beating.

Then came the finding that an old manual method developed by Kouwenhoven, the engineer who had introduced defibrillation, could help. He had shown that a person whose heart has stopped beating can be kept alive by compressing the lower part of the breastbone rhythmically. Such compression moved enough blood to keep alive the heart, brain and other vital organs. It provided time to get equipment to the patient's bedside.

But it was the special coronary care unit that was to make the big difference. Here, as we have noted and shall see in more detail in Chapter 17, the equipment is right at hand. Defibrillation can be started immediately; there is no delay. In a coronary care unit, there is constant monitoring of the patient's heart functioning. Nurses in a coronary care unit are trained to recognize dangerous abnormal rhythms and have the authority to start lifesaving treatment, if necessary, without awaiting the arrival of a physician.

In the beginning, coronary care units focused on resuscitation, and thus saved many lives. If a patient could be treated within one minute after his heart went into fibrillation, he had a 90 percent or even better chance to live. If there were a three-minute delay, he had a 10 percent chance. In a coronary care unit, he could be treated within a minute.

Then came another major development—the use of the unit to *prevent* fibrillation. Ventricular fibrillation develops suddenly— but is, it was found, almost invariably preceded by other abnormal rhythms. These rhythms could be detected. And they could be treated so that fibrillation would not follow. It was found that an excellent drug for such treatment is lidocaine, the compound commonly used by dentists as a local anesthetic. It can be infused continuously into a vein in tiny amounts for forty-eight hours or longer until the abnormal rhythms disappear. In hospitals where reviews have been made of carefully kept long-term records, it has been found that where once 15 percent of heart-attack patients developed ventricular fibrillation, now less than 1 percent do.

Thus, in very recent years, there has been a great change in the outlook for heart-attack victims—for those who get to the hospital in time to benefit not only from immediate treatment but also from the monitoring and precautionary measures which are now available to treat and even avoid serious electrical disturbances of the heart.

[14]

Preventive Measures

What provokes coronary heart disease? Perhaps no other aspect of modern medicine has led to so much public confusion as the search for the possible causes of the corrosion that affects the inner surfaces of the coronary arteries and may eventually lead to heart attack.

It would be nice if there were some single, readily remedial cause, as some reports published in the past have seemed to suggest. But the best medical minds are convinced that many factors are involved rather than just one.

Cholesterol has been blamed for years. This soft, waxy, yellowish substance comes from a variety of foods. It is also produced in the body by the liver. It circulates through the blood stream.

A statistical correlation between abnormally high levels of cholesterol in the blood and coronary heart disease has been established by dozens of studies. Investigations have also shown that blood cholesterol can be lowered by dietary means and that when it is lowered there is a reduction in the incidence of heart attacks.

One study conducted by physicians at the Atherosclerosis Re-

167

search Center in Montclair, New Jersey, covered 200 men, aged twenty to fifty, over a five-year period. All had had heart attacks. One hundred were placed on a diet aimed at reducing cholesterol levels. The other hundred were allowed to eat anything they liked. At the end of the five years, the men in the unrestricted diet group had a heart-attack recurrence rate 150 percent greater than the other men did.

But if cholesterol is involved in heart disease, it is also obvious that so are other factors. Not long ago, scientists discovered the town of Roseto, Pennsylvania, whose 1,630 inhabitants, largely of Italian descent, love prosciuto (pressed ham with an inch of fat on it), fried peppers and bread dipped in lard gravy. Their whole way of life goes against calorie-counting and fat-watching. Their average daily caloric intake, above the national average, is 3,000 for men, 2,300 for women, and most of the calories come from fat.

Yet Rosetans have only one-third the heart-attack rate of people in surrounding areas. Medical teams, examining the townspeople, have found that their average blood cholesterol level is the same as that of other people who have three times greater heart-attack incidence.

What accounts for the heart health of Rosetans? It may be their sensible way of life, the investigators who came to study them believe. "The most striking feature of Roseto," investigating physicians have reported, "was the way in which people seemed to enjoy life. They were gay, boisterous, unpretentious . . . simple, warm and very hospitable . . . mutually trusting (there is no crime in Roseto) and mutually supporting. There is poverty but no real want, since neighbors provide for the needy."

American scientists have gone to Africa to study Masai tribesmen, trying to discover why these herdsmen and warriors never seem to get heart trouble in spite of a diet containing enough cholesterol to send Americans fleeing in panic from the dinner table.

The Masai live almost exclusively on meat and milk with a butterfat content that soars to 6.5 percent. Yet they have far lower blood cholesterol levels on the average than Americans.

Was it exercise that protected Masai arteries, keeping cholesterol levels in the blood low despite huge intake? The Masai are known to walk as much as 60 miles a day without strain. The scientists took along a treadmill that moves at 1½ miles per hour and tilts progressively upward at the front end, 1 degree a minute, making it increasingly difficult to keep walking or even stay on it.

Where the average healthy U.S. college boy lasts 14 minutes before being spilled off the back end, exhausted and gasping for breath, some of the Masai walked the treadmill through its maximum scale of thirty minutes and 30-degree elevation. Even old men lasted twenty minutes and longer, and not one sat down afterward.

Yet exercise did not appear to be the whole answer to the Masai mystery, for it turned out that the Masai have much less heart disease than neighboring tribes who are just as active physically.

More recently, two American pathologists who lived among the Masai and examined them thoroughly reported what they believe to be the reason: The Masai seem to have a special genetic endowment. Their livers and intestines, unlike those of Americans and of others, do not convert much of the cholesterol they eat into the kind of fat that is deposited on the lining of blood vessels. (Cholesterol-rich foods contain large molecules of cholesterol. Several organs of the body, but mainly the liver, change this cholesterol into smaller molecules of beta lipoproteins, which are more easily transported in the blood and deposited in artery walls.)

The Masai appear to have a remarkable mechanism that makes only so many beta lipoproteins and no more, no matter how much cholesterol they eat. When, for example, the two pathologists set up an experiment in which twenty-four tribesmen ate a normal Masai diet and twelve of the twenty-four were given two extra grams a day of cholesterol, the two groups were found to have almost exactly the same levels of fats in the blood.

But if exercise does not seem to be the reason for the Masai's relative imperviousness to coronary heart disease, evidence of the protective value of exercise has come from many other studies. In London, England, conductors who climb the stairs of double-decker buses to collect fares have a much lower heart-disease rate than inactive bus drivers have. University of Minnesota investigators, studying the records of more than 200,000 American railroad workers, found that desk-bound clerks have twice the heart-attack rate of section hands, whose jobs are more strenuous.

Harvard scientists, comparing 700 Boston men of Irish descent, aged thirty to sixty, with their brothers who stayed in Ireland, found the heart-disease death rate twice as high in the Boston group. Although the men in Ireland ate more eggs, butter and other saturated fats, they had lower cholesterol levels. And although they consumed 400 calories more per day than their Boston brothers, they weighed 10 percent less. The men in Ireland get more exercise, and their lower cholesterol levels show that physical activity does more than burn off calories.

According to a study of 55,000 men covered by the Health Insurance Plan of New York, if a man leads a physically active life, he not only has a far better chance of escaping a heart attack but also has as much as a three-times-greater chance of surviving one than a less active man.

Regular exercise provides training for the heart muscle, enabling it to perform more effectively under all circumstances, including physical and mental stress. It may help another way as well, stimulating the build-up of smaller vessels, collaterals, to take the place of narrowed channels or to bypass points of narrowing.

Stress appears to be another major influence in the development of coronary trouble. One of many studies indicating this was carried out by Dr. Henry I. Russek, a New York heart specialist, who analyzed the histories of one hundred young coronary patients. He found that ninety-one of the one hundred had been under severe stress—working more than sixty hours a week or experiencing unusual fear, insecurity, discontent, restlessness or feelings of inadequacy in relation to employment.

Dr. Russek also checked on 12,000 professional men and found a striking correlation between job stress and coronary disease. For example, the coronary-disease rate was three to four times greater among general practitioners of medicine, dentistry and law than among specialists in the same professions, who may work under somewhat less strain.

What of excessive smoking? For twenty years, Framingham,

Massachusetts, has been a special place. National Heart Institute investigators have been following 5,000 residents of that town, aged thirty to sixty, in an intensive effort to plumb the factors in coronary disease. Excessive smoking appears to be a major factor. Smokers of two packs of cigarettes a day had an incidence of sudden death from heart attacks five times greater than that of nonsmokers. Framingham investigators made a hopeful discovery: heavy smokers who gave up smoking had thereafter about the same incidence of heart attacks as men who had never smoked.

The Framingham study has been showing, as have many other studies, that elevated blood pressure, diabetes, gout and emotional stress are all contributing factors in heart attacks.

Thus a composite picture of many risk factors in coronary heart disease has emerged. It is not yet possible to have a full view of their relative importance and interaction. There are many gaps in our knowledge.

But even as research to close the gaps goes forward, there are valuable guidelines which can be put to use.

LESSENING THE RISK

Let us consider, on a realistic basis, just what can be done about minimizing these risk factors: what your physician can help accomplish and what you can do for yourself.

Hypertension

High blood pressure seems to have a considerable effect on atherosclerosis of the coronary arteries, the clogging that sets the stage for a heart attack. Hypertension and atherosclerosis very often go together. Among people with uncontrolled hypertension, coronary heart disease is the most common cause of death. And experimental studies with animals have shown hypertension to have definite effects on the development and progression of atherosclerosis.

The exact mechanism by which hypertension promotes

atherosclerosis still is not clear. For one thing, blood-pressure elevation seems to affect the lipid profile—the types and amounts of fats in the blood—adversely. It has also been suggested that hypertension increases pressure against the inner lining of the coronary arteries, enabling fat-containing substances to enter it.

As we explained earlier (see Chapter 6), if you have hypertension you are not likely to discover the fact for yourself. Your physician will most likely find it during the course of a routine examination. And, as we said, it is now possible to control hypertension, even the most severe kind, in the vast majority of cases. Mild hypertension can often be controlled by changes in diet and in salt intake. Or suitable drug treatment can bring down pressure.

It is therefore wise and practical for you to be on guard against hypertension and its effects on the coronary arteries by having regular periodic examinations. If hypertension should be found, you should allow your physician to begin suitable treatment without delay.

Diabetes

A high incidence of atherosclerosis is associated with diabetes. The artery disease appears to develop much more frequently, at an earlier age and in more severe form in diabetic persons than in the general population. The likelihood of death from heart attack is more than twice as great for the diabetic.

Establishing the exact role of diabetes in atherosclerosis is complicated, because there is a high incidence of hypertension and also of obesity among diabetics—and both of these of themselves are, of course, factors in atherosclerosis. It is known, however, that great changes in lipid metabolism—the way the body handles fats—occur when a diabetic passes from good control of his diabetes to inadequate control. And so, if you happen to have diabetes, it is vital that you maintain good control of it and that you have routine periodic checks to make certain that the control is good.

Gout

When the body burns its fuels—fats, carbohydrates and proteins—certain waste products are produced. One of these is uric acid. If, through an imbalance in the system, excess uric acid accumulates, gout often appears. Gout may affect the joints. It frequently starts with attacks of very severe pain in one joint, often the big toe. It is much more common in men than in women. And when gout is present, the coronary arteries are more likely to become prematurely diseased.

But excess levels of uric acid may be present without producing the symptoms of gout. It would appear to be the excess levels, with or without the gout symptoms, which influence coronary heart disease. It has been suggested that uric acid acts as a conditioning agent on artery linings, enhancing the deposit of fatty substances.

There are simple tests to detect excess uric acid. And today there are very effective measures for controlling gout and reducing uric-acid levels to normal. In some milder cases, moderation of diet alone may be enough. In others, medication may be used.

Thus, if you have gout, you don't have to go on experiencing attacks. And the bringing down of excess uric-acid levels will help, too, to reduce your risk of coronary heart disease. If you do not have gout symptoms but your physician discovers excess uric acid levels, you will now appreciate his reason for recommending diet or medication to return the levels to normal.

Low Thyroid-Gland Function

Hypothyroidism, or underfunctioning of the thyroid gland, is associated with elevated fat levels in the blood. The thyroid secretes a hormone which in part controls the way cholesterol is excreted from the body.

Any of several tests can be used to verify the presence of hypothyroidism when it is suspected, and thyroid medication can be used to counteract the problem—and, at the same time, to reduce the level of blood fats.

Smoking

As early as the turn of the century, the fact that smoking, particularly cigarette smoking, exerted stress on blood vessels, narrowing the caliber of arteries, became apparent in a condition called Buerger's disease. Patients who have this problem of the leg arteries experience cramping and severe pain of the leg muscles when they walk. In those patients who persisted in smoking, the disease usually progressed to the point of gangrene and made amputation necessary.

Later it was noted that, in some patients with coronary heart disease and angina pectoris, smoking could trigger an attack of chest pain. It seemed that certain individuals were particularly sensitive to tobacco.

But it has only been in recent years that the significant role of cigarette smoking in heart disease has been established.

Many studies have demonstrated that freedom from coronary atherosclerosis is much more common in nonsmokers than in smokers. Moreover, the extent of the atherosclerosis in smokers has been found to increase with the number of cigarettes smoked daily.

Investigations by Dr. Charles W. Frank and his associates of 110,000 adults enrolled in the Health Insurance Plan of Greater New York revealed that previously healthy men and women who smoke cigarettes run twice the risk of a heart attack that nonsmokers do.

Other studies have shown that nonsmokers face only a fifth the risk of dying suddenly from a first heart attack, compared with smokers of one pack a day or more. Recently Dr. David Spain of Brooklyn and his associates reported on the postmortem examination of 291 subjects who had died suddenly of coronary heart disease. They found that heavy smokers survived a shorter time after the attack and were an average of sixteen years younger than the nonsmokers.

It now seems clear that cigarette smoking contributes both to the development of coronary heart disease and to death from it, although some predisposing factor such as excessive levels of blood fat may be necessary. The entire mechanism by which smoking exerts its effects is still not entirely clear, but some factors are known.

Smoking causes an increase in the heart rate. It also produces a temporary rise in blood pressure. A recent study has shown that smoking even a low-nicotine filter cigarette raises systolic blood pressure by 8 points and produces a nine-beat-a-minute increase in heart rate. Other studies have shown that cigarette smoking stimulates the release of hormones from the adrenal gland which have powerful effects on the heart and circulation and influence the levels of fats circulating in the blood stream.

Another recent study indicates that the red blood cells of smokers have less affinity for oxygen. As much as 20 percent of the blood being pushed around by the heart of the smoker is not working so far as carrying oxygen is concerned. Since the heart has the highest oxygen requirement per unit weight of any tissue, any change in the supply of oxygen could affect the heart first and thereby increase the risk of an attack for the smoker.

As far as heart disease is concerned, there is a distinct difference between cigarette smoking and pipe or cigar smoking. A possible explanation is that a cigar smoker does not usually inhale, and even if he does he seldom inhales as deeply as the cigarette smoker. That is equally true for the pipe smoker—who in addition may spend proportionately less time smoking because of the time he spends tamping, packing, lighting and relighting his pipe.

Based on all the evidence, then, giving up cigarette smoking is, to put it mildly, a wise move.

If you are not now a smoker, don't begin. If you are a cigarette smoker, even though you may have made abortive attempts to quit the habit in the past, you may be more successful now. A considerable number of people—including a great many doctors— have shown that it can be done. If there is a stop-smoking clinic in your community, you may find it worthwhile to attend. Your physician will have other suggestions to help you break the habit.

If your urge to smoke is so strong that you cannot resist, we would strongly advise that you try switching to pipes or cigars.

Excessive Weight

Many studies have shown that excessive weight increases the risk of coronary heart disease. In the Government's Framingham study, for example, men who were 30 percent overweight were 2.8 times as likely to develop coronary heart disease in ten years as were men who were 10 percent or more underweight. Particularly marked in the overweight group was the likelihood of developing angina pectoris.

Excess weight may promote coronary heart disease by placing an added work load on the heart. Also, in many cases the person who is overweight has elevated blood pressure. And blood fat abnormalities are more common in the overweight.

Happily, weight reduction is accompanied by a decrease in mortality risk and by improvement in blood-pressure and blood-fat levels.

Are You Overweight?   By definition, an obese person is anyone who weighs 30 percent or more over what he or she should weigh. Even if you are not that much overweight, it can be important to lose the first 10 pounds of excess. The odds are that if you are overweight at all you will gain more in the future, and it is easier to lose 10 pounds than to lose 20 or 30 pounds—or more.

Your mirror can provide a fairly good indication of whether you are too heavy. If you think that your eyes deceive you, you can consult the accompanying table:

Unlike some other tables, this one provides *desirable* rather than *average* weights. Average people tend to become fat over the years, and average weight tables reflect the fat people who make up the upper part of the average.

There are also simple tests you can use to help assess your actual fatness.

DESIRABLE WEIGHTS FOR MEN AND WOMEN

(Weight in pounds, according to frame, as ordinarily dressed, including shoes)

MEN

Height (with shoes on) Feet	Inches	Small Frame	Medium Frame	Large Frame
5	2	116–125	124–133	131–142
5	3	119–128	127–136	133–144
5	4	122–132	130–140	137–149
5	5	126–136	134–144	141–153
5	6	129–139	137–147	145–157
5	7	133–143	141–151	149–162
5	8	136–147	145–160	153–166
5	9	140–151	149–160	157–170
5	10	144–155	153–164	161–175
5	11	148–164	157–168	165–180
6	0	152–164	161–173	168–185
6	1	157–169	166–178	174–190
6	2	163–175	171–184	179–196
6	3	168–180	176–189	184–202

WOMEN

Height (with shoes on) Feet	Inches	Small Frame	Medium Frame	Large Frame
4	11	104–111	110–118	117–127
5	0	105–113	112–120	119–129
5	1	107–115	114–122	121–131
5	2	110–118	117–125	124–135
5	3	113–121	120–128	127–138
5	4	116–125	124–132	131–142
5	5	119–128	127–135	133–145
5	6	123–132	130–140	138–150
5	7	126–136	134–144	142–154
5	8	129–139	137–147	145–158
5	9	133–143	141–151	149–162
5	10	136–147	145–155	152–166
5	11	139–150	148–158	155–169

The *ruler* test is based on the fact that the abdominal surface between the flare of the ribs and front of the pelvis normally is flat if there is no excess fat present. Lie flat on your back and place a ruler on your abdomen, along the midline of the body. The ruler should not point upward at the midsection. If it does, it indicates a need to slim down.

The *pinch* or *skinfold* test calls for grasping a "pinch" of skin with your thumb and forefinger at your side, abdomen, upper arm, buttocks and calf. At least half of body fat is directly under the skin. The layer beneath the skin—which is what you measure when you pinch—should be between one-fourth and one-half inch thick. When you pinch, you are getting a double thickness. If the fold is much greater than an inch thick it indicates excess fatness.

Reducing: The Fad Diets.   At any one time, 20 million people in this country are on some reducing diet or other. Dieting has come to be the Number One national pastime.

Fad diets have become big business. They are incredibly numerous. Many, if not most, are self-defeating, and some are actually health-impairing.

There are crash diets which focus on grapefruit and coffee for days on end, or celery and virtually nothing else. The idea seems to be to put up with being miserable in the hope that a lot of fat can be melted away in a short time. But acute malnutrition may develop. And there have been fatalities from crash diets.

There are low-carbohydrate diets which restrict "carbohydrate unit" intake but allow just about anything else. There are high-protein diets which restrict intake to steak, eggs and other high-protein foods. There are even "eat fat" diets which supposedly put the fats you eat to work by somehow melting away fat deposits in the body.

Any single-category diet can be dangerous because it omits other necessary food groups. A diet high in fats may actually add to the danger of coronary heart disease.

Even when they are not clearly dangerous, fad diets are self-defeating. They may appear to be initially successful, but the weight loss may be from water rather than body fat. Even when there is fat loss, the fat is quickly regained because once the diet is over, there is usually a quick return to the original faulty eating habits which led to the excess weight in the first place.

Actually, there is evidence that frequent ups and downs in weight may be more harmful than maintaining a steady excess weight. If you go on a crash diet and do take off weight, and then, after the diet is over, put on weight again, and sooner or later go on another diet, with the same end results, your blood cholesterol level will rise during each period of weight gain, thus increasing the risk that fats will be deposited on the artery walls. There is no evidence to show that once fats are deposited they can be removed by weight reduction.

There have been animal studies showing that normal-weight animals have longer life expectancy than obese animals—and these studies have also shown that obese animals subjected to repeated weight losses and gains have even shorter life expectancies than obese animals that have never reduced.

Reducing: The Right Way. The principles for taking off excess weight—and keeping it off—are not complicated.

If you eat more calories than your body uses up, you gain weight. If your caloric intake is less than your caloric expenditure, you lose weight. If you are to lose one pound of fat, you must use up 3,500 more calories than you eat.

It is helpful, as we have noted previously, to increase your physical activity as a means of aiding in weight reduction.

Coupled with this, you need a sound reducing diet. That means it should produce weight loss at a safe pace. At the same time, it should offer variety, a balance of foods, to maintain health. And, fully as important, it should teach new and enjoyable eating patterns so you do not promptly revert to old, weight-gaining eating habits.

Moreover, today it makes sense that a reducing diet be consistent with changes in the American diet which are being advocated by many physicians and by health organizations such as the American Heart Association. These are changes in the direction of modifying fat intake to reduce the risk of atherosclerosis.

Although the cause of coronary atherosclerosis is not definitely known, we do know some of the factors involved.

For example, we believe that a metabolic error involving the body's ability to handle fat is in part responsible for the build-up of deposits that narrow the coronary arteries. Some of the fat involved—about one-third of it—comes from food; the remainder is produced within the body.

The food fats believed to lead to atherosclerosis are the so-called saturated fats contained in dairy products, meats and various natural oils. We ask patients to reduce the total quantity of saturated fats ingested to about one-half of what is contained in the ordinary American diet. This requires less intake of such common items as butter, whole milk, cheeses and other dairy products as well as a sharp reduction in the total quantity of meat which has a large content of saturated fat even when it is lean. A single *ounce* of steak, for example, contains 5 grams of fat, the amount found in a *pound* of filet of sole.

In the Appendix is an overall fat-controlled meal plan prepared by, and published through the courtesy of, the American Heart Association. This plan can be helpful to you and your whole family even if none of you needs to lose weight. But if you do need to control your weight, you will find the plan valuable for its suggested limitations on sizes of servings and on fat in particular. If you need a vigorous weight-reduction plan, you can work one out with your physician, using the plan in the Appendix as a base.

Your physician may, if he thinks it suitable for you, prescribe a a booklet published by the American Heart Association, called *Planning Fat-Controlled Meals for 1200 and 1800 Calories*. The booklet, which is available only on a physician's prescription, makes use of the same principles as those shown in the plan in the Appendix. It provides sample menus for both 1,200- and 1,800-calorie diets and also offers useful recipes.

High Cholesterol

As far back as 1908, a Russian investigator, Ignatowski, was able to demonstrate that the feeding of eggs to rabbits led to development of atherosclerosis. Ever since, there has been agreement that the feeding of cholesterol elevates levels of cholesterol, a fatlike substance in the blood, and causes atherosclerosis in experimental animals. Many hundreds of experiments have been carried out with chickens, rabbits, guinea pigs, mice, pigs and monkeys.

Evidence associating cholesterol in the diet with coronary heart disease has come from studies of various population groups which indicate that this disease is rare when a given population, such as the Japanese, eat a diet low in fat and cholesterol. On the other hand, coronary heart disease is common in peoples of North America and Europe, who commonly consume the high-cholesterol, high-fat American type of diet.

As evidence accumulated indicating that cholesterol in the blood stream might be deposited in artery walls, it seemed logical to try to reduce the levels of cholesterol in the blood by reducing the dietary intake of cholesterol. But it soon developed that merely restricting cholesterol intake did not markedly reduce blood cholesterol levels.

The next step was the discovery that the amount of fats in the diet mattered. Individuals on a low-cholesterol diet but a diet still high in fats continued to have elevated cholesterol levels. A considerable amount of research was needed to clear up the puzzle.

Fat in the diet was found to facilitate the absorption of cholesterol from food. The body produces cholesterol, which is secreted in bile which flows into the intestinal tract. But with fat in the intestine, cholesterol from bile was reabsorbed instead of being eliminated.

Still, when a low-fat diet was tried, it did not always lead to blood cholesterol reduction. Could it be the type of fat that was important? That, indeed, proved to be the case.

The Differences in Fats. There are several distinctive types of fats.

Saturated fats are the type that tend to raise the level of cholesterol in the blood. These are fats that harden at room temperature, such as the fat in gravy. They are found, as we have seen, in most animal products and some hydrogenated vegetable products.

Saturated animal fats occur in beef, lamb, pork and ham; in

butter, cream and whole milk; and in cheeses made from cream and whole milk.

Saturated vegetable fats are found in many solid and hydrogenated shortenings, and in the coconut oil, cocoa butter and palm oil used in commercially prepared cookies, pie fillings and non-dairy milk and cream substitutes.

Polyunsaturated fats tend to lower blood cholesterol levels by helping to eliminate excess, newly formed cholesterol. These are fats which tend to remain liquid at room temperature. They are usually liquid oils of vegetable origin. Oils such as corn, cottonseed, safflower, sesame seed, soybean, and sunflower seed are high in polyunsaturated fat.

By reducing the amount of saturated fats and cholesterol in the diet, you can lower blood cholesterol. If you substitute some polyunsaturated fats for the saturated type, blood cholesterol comes down further.

Mono-unsaturated fats are a third type. They appear to have little effect on blood cholesterol. Olive oil is one example.

Here's a quick lesson in the chemistry of fats: A saturated type is one containing all the hydrogen atoms it can hold. A polyunsaturated type has room to add four or more hydrogen atoms and thus change to a saturated fat. A mono-unsaturated fat can hold two more hydrogen atoms. For many years, hydrogenation—the addition of hydrogen atoms—was used with some oils to produce margarines and vegetable shortenings. Today, while there are still completely hydrogenated oils, most margarines and shortenings contain partially hydrogenated oils plus acceptable amounts of polyunsaturates.

Actually, no food is made up completely of any one type of fat. Foods vary in their proportions of all three types.

Foods high in saturated fats include cream, butter, lard, eggs, cheeses, meats, chocolate and coconut oil. These foods have relatively few polyunsaturated fats. Next in order come vegetable shortenings and margarines, which generally have about half of the saturated fats found in meat or dairy fat.

Foods highest in polyunsaturated fats and lowest in saturates include liquid vegetable oils which have not been hydrogenated, and liquid shortenings made of lightly hydrogenated vegetable oils. Also in this group belong the newer margarines.

Corn, cottonseed and soya oils contain about 55 percent poly-unsaturated fats, 10 to 25 percent saturated fats and the remainder mono-unsaturated. Butter contains about 50 percent saturated fat and less than 10 percent polyunsaturated, with the rest consisting of mono-unsaturated.

Cholesterol is present in moderate amounts in all animal tissues. It occurs, for example, in fat-containing dairy products and the muscle meat of beef, pork, poultry, fish and seafood. It is present in higher amounts in such organ meats as liver and kidney. And it is especially high in a few foods, such as egg yolks and brains.

A Fat-Controlled, Low-Cholesterol Diet. For some years, there has been controversy over the need to make a broad-scale recommendation for a change in the eating habits of millions of people.

We still do not know the exact role of elevated blood cholesterol levels in the development of atherosclerosis and coronary heart disease. Nor are we certain exactly how much good reduction of these levels will do to prevent the development or progression of coronary heart disease. To determine this will take several decades of observation of the effects on large numbers of people.

Nevertheless, there is enough evidence that high cholesterol levels do contribute to the development of atherosclerosis to make more and more physicians and health authorities urge action now against the risks that millions of us are taking.

Moreover, this nutritional action is practical, for it involves moderate rather than drastic changes in diet. You do not have to give up all your favorite dishes and can still enjoy your mealtimes. As you will note from the plan in the Appendix, there is room for variety and for many of the foods you undoubtedly relish.

As the American Heart Association explains, the plan has four goals: (1) to meet your daily need for essential nutrients, including protein, vitamins and minerals; (2) to control calories and maintain a desirable weight; (3) to avoid excessive amounts of saturated fat and cholesterol by lowering your intake of foods particularly rich in them; and (4) to see that more of the fat you eat is polyunsaturated, and less of it is saturated.

To control your intake of cholesterol-rich foods requires that you (1) eat no more than three egg yolks a week, including eggs used in cooking, and (2) limit your use of shellfish and organ meats.

To control the amount and type of fat you eat requires that you (1) use fish, chicken, turkey and veal in most of your meat meals for the week, and limit beef, lamb, pork and ham to five moderate-sized portions per week; (2) choose lean cuts of meat, trim any visible fat and discard any fat that cooks out of the meat; (3) avoid deep-fat frying and use cooking methods that help to remove fat—baking, boiling, broiling, roasting, stewing; (4) restrict your use of fatty "luncheon" and "variety" meats such as sausages and salami; (5) use liquid vegetable oils and margarines rich in polyunsaturated fats in place of butter and other cooking fats that are solid or completely hydrogenated; (6) use skimmed milk and skimmed-milk cheeses in place of whole milk and cheeses made from whole milk and cream.

Another Fat Problem—Triglycerides

Cholesterol is only one of the fatty materials—called lipids—found in the blood. Triglycerides—glycerines combined with three fatty acids—are actually the main form in which fats appear in the body.

Elevation of cholesterol levels without elevation of triglycerides is most common. In some people, however, the levels of triglycerides are markedly elevated and are believed to play a role in atherosclerosis.

Abnormally high triglyceride levels are often associated with obesity, excessive intake of carbohydrates (sugars and starches), diabetes, alcoholism, underfunctioning of the thyroid gland, kidney disease and, in some women, the use of estrogens, as in oral contraceptives. In obese patients, high triglyceride levels can often be lowered by weight reduction alone. In other cases, a specific diet defect must be corrected.

When a diet rich in carbohydrates is the cause, for example, reduction of carbohydrate intake in addition to use of unsaturated fats with a minimum of saturated fats can be effective.

Drugs That Reduce Cholesterol and Triglycerides. If diet and the other measures we have discussed fail to bring down elevated levels of cholesterol or triglycerides adequately, a drug may be used to help.

One of the most useful drugs is clofibrate. It is effective in reducing elevated triglycerides, although how it does so is unknown. It is also considered by many physicians to be the most useful of available drugs for reducing elevated cholesterol levels. Clofibrate both inhibits the body's manufacture of cholesterol and increases its excretion from the body. Along with clofibrate, dietary measures are also essential, and in some patients it may be necessary to use sodium dextrothyroxine or sitosterols as well. Sodium dextrothyroxine is often effective in lowering cholesterol, although, again, the mechanism of its action is not known. Sitosterols act to lower cholesterol by interfering with intestinal absorption of cholesterol from both food and bile.

Emotional Stress

As we have said, scientists have found that emotional stress may promote heart attacks. For example, the rate of coronary heart disease among security traders on the New York Stock Exchange was found to be more than twice as great as that among security analysts, who presumably do less stressful work.

It has been shown that heart rate and blood pressure will generally rise markedly during periods of stress. In addition, stress may increase blood cholesterol levels. Dr. Meyer Friedman and Dr. Ray H. Rosenman of Mount Zion Hospital and Medical Center, San Francisco, studied a group of forty certified public accountants between the ages of thirty-five and sixty and found that their average cholesterol level rose from 210 to 252 milligrams per hundred cubic centimeters of blood in periods of greatest stress, such as shortly before tax deadlines. Also, their blood tended to clot more rapidly in periods of maximum stress. Other scientists have reported similar findings in studies of medical students immediately before final examinations.

Some investigators emphasize that it is not so much the stress itself which is important but rather the individual's response to stress. All of us are subjected to stress of one kind or another, but we do not all respond alike to it. To a large degree, response depends on an individual's basic personality.

There have been intensive efforts to focus on how specific personality patterns may influence proneness to coronary heart disease. Dr. Friedman and Dr. Rosenman in San Francisco began in 1960 to study the effects of personality among 3,411 men, aged thirty-nine to fifty-nine, working for eleven California corporations. They found that the person most likely to experience a heart attack is the hard-driving man who is intensely competitive and obsessively ambitious, and constantly battling deadlines.

Among the first sixty-nine men from this group who suffered heart attacks, 73 percent had previously been diagnosed as being prone to coronary heart disease on the basis of these personality characteristics.

The work of Dr. Friedman and Dr. Rosenman indicates that perhaps half of all individuals have such personality characteristics, whether they are white-collar or blue-collar workers, clerks or executives. To a greater or lesser extent, they are afflicted by a sense of urgency. Always unsatisfied, they try to squeeze in more and more activities in given periods of time.

"They sometimes go to almost ludicrous limits to accomplish this squeezing in of events," Dr. Friedman has noted. "For example, some subjects like to evacuate their bowels, read the financial section of the newspaper and shave with an electric razor all at the same time. One subject admitted that he had already purchased ten different electric razors in his efforts to find one that would shave faster than all others, and another subject liked to use two electric razors at the same time so that he could cut his shaving time in half.

"This harrowing sense of time urgency," Dr. Friedman notes further, "can be detected by questions dealing with (1) his punctuality (he is always punctual), (2) his attitude about waiting for a table in a restaurant (he never will wait if he can possibly avoid it), (3) his attitude toward persons who take quite a long time to come to a point in conversation (he will try to bring them quickly to the point or begin to think of some other subject which truly interests him). But the simplest way of detecting this sense of time urgency is for the interviewer himself to begin to ask a question (whose answer is obvious to the interviewee before the question is completed) and then begin to stutter before the entire question has been asked. Invariably the interviewee will burst in and answer the question as the interviewer is still attempting to stutter out its end."

We cannot avoid stress. By our reactions to stress, we can accentuate its influence. It is difficult, though not impossible, to change personality characteristics. We may be helped to some degree in making at least partial favorable modifications by an understanding of our characteristics—a real awareness that we have them and an insight into their adverse effects.

There is something more we can do about mental and emotional stress. We may be able to mitigate the effects by resorting to physical activity. Very probably, you have more than once had the experience of being extremely tense, caught up in some problem, worrying and anxious about it, unable at the moment to see a solution—and of finding it difficult to sit still. Your body seemed to be crying out for movement. You may have gotten up and paced the room.

At moments of stress, physical activity may serve as an escape valve. It is a good idea for all of us to have some form of regular physical activity as a kind of antidote for mental and emotional stress. Some investigators have suggested that with stress there is an outpouring of hormones from the adrenal glands, the hormones intended to ready the body for activity. Without the activity, substances derived from these hormones may accumulate in the heart and over a long period of time affect heart function. With physical activity, such substances may be destroyed and further accumulations may be prevented.

A CALL FOR EXERCISE

As we have seen, exercise correctly used may help to prevent a heart attack or, if a heart attack does occur, to improve your chances of surviving it.

But exercise is not a panacea. For coronary heart disease, there *is* no panacea. Since many factors appear to be involved in the development of coronary atherosclerosis, even the most scrupulous attention to one factor will not assure that the disease will be prevented.

Still, properly used, exercise can be an important aid for the health of the heart and circulation and of the body in general.

Most of us today live soft, sedentary lives. Almost every so-called modern advance—power tools, automation, elevators, automobiles, TV sets, even electric toothbrushes—contributes to a progressive reduction in physical activity.

Evidence that inadequate physical activity promotes coronary heart disease has been marshaled from many studies. Some of these we described at the beginning of this chapter. Among others is a study by Harold A. Kahn of the National Heart Institute of more than 2,000 Post Office workers in Washington, D.C. It showed that the risk of developing coronary heart disease was as much as 1.9 times greater among the clerks than it was among the mail carriers.

Dr. Daniel Brunner of Israel's Tel Aviv University has studied coronary heart disease among more than 10,000 sedentary and nonsedentary workers in Israeli kibbutzim (collective settlements). Over a fifteen-year period, the death rate was as much as four times greater among the sedentary workers.

As we have noted, some studies indicate that exercise tends to reduce the risk of coronary heart disease by helping the body to maintain normal cholesterol levels despite relatively high intakes of fat. Exercise also contributes to weight reduction and to reduction of elevated blood pressure.

Vanderbilt University investigators carried out a study with a group of men, twenty-one to forty years of age. Each man had at least one coronary disease contributory factor present: high cholesterol, obesity or hypertension. Some had two factors; a few had three. The men undertook a six-week conditioning program, beginning with mild calisthenics and building up to mile-long runs. There was no prescribed diet; each man ate as he pleased. By the end of the program, average weight loss was six pounds, and cholesterol and blood-pressure levels were markedly lower.

At the University of Oregon Medical School, investigators fed radioactively tagged cholesterol to animals. By the tagging, they could follow what happened to the cholesterol. They found that the more the animals exercised, the more cholesterol was broken down; the less exercise, the higher the levels of cholesterol in the blood.

The contribution of exercise to reduction of excessive weight is considerable and often not fully appreciated. Physical activity requires energy, and energy requires calories. At first glance, the amount of activity needed to use up the 3,500 calories in a pound of body fat may seem formidable. It appears discouraging that a 150-pound person, walking at a rate of 3 miles an hour, will have to walk for an hour just to use up 240 calories. Yet, if he walks only half an hour a day and does not increase the amount of calories he takes in, he can expect to lose over twelve pounds in a year.

And, as we have seen, exercise can have a conditioning effect on the heart. When you are at rest, body muscles use only about 1/30 of the oxygen they use during maximum effort. With exercise, as they need more oxygen, the heart responds by pumping harder to get more oxygen-carrying blood into circulation. As a result, over a period of time the heart's pumping efficiency tends to increase. The heart becomes able to pump more blood with each stroke.

Investigators have reported that the trained or conditioned heart may become so much more efficient that when the body is at rest it will beat more slowly, function more economically and require less oxygen for a given amount of work. Moreover, the well-conditioned body itself requires a smaller amount of heart-muscle activity for any given physical performance.

As one investigator puts it, "Physical activity is a form of training that permits the heart to adjust more readily to periods of stress." This appears to be true even for the stress of an actual heart attack. For exercise increases the blood supply to the heart by increasing the network of blood vessels feeding the heart. Thus, if a blood clot should shut off one of the coronary artery branches, the effect on the heart would be much less damaging.

Proper exercise, then, is beneficial; we underscore *proper* because improper exercise can be dangerous, even deadly. Rush in without preparation and try to lift 200 pounds above your head, or run 2 miles, or play several sets of tennis, and it may be your last act on earth. It is absolutely essential that exercise be approached gingerly; that it be started at a reasonable, comfortable level; that it be increased gradually.

Exercise at Any Age. There is a common misconception that anyone beyond the age of forty is too old to exercise. This, of course, is belied by many older people who engage in vigorous exercise regularly without difficulty. They may not have the same stamina they had when they were eighteen, but they have far more stamina than many overfed, underexercised contemporary eighteen-year-olds.

Studies show that elderly people can regain much of the vigor of their earlier years through carefully planned physical activity. A University of Southern California investigation covered sixty-nine men, aged fifty to eighty-seven. For a period of a year, beginning very slowly and progressing gradually, working out three times a week for an hour at a time, they did calisthenics, stretching exercises, swimming and jogging. At the end of the year, these were the results expressed in terms of group averages: blood pressure reduced by 6 percent; body fat decreased by 4.8 percent; arm strength increased by 7.2 percent. Nervous tension was also reduced.

If you have been ill or if you have a heart condition, you should check with your physician before undertaking any program of physical activity. He can advise you about how to proceed. It is also worth consulting him even if you do not have a heart or other problem.

Generally, the best way to get started is by walking. Walking brings into play many muscles. It is a continuous type of activity. It lends itself to a slow start and a gradual build-up in physical effort.

You can begin with a ten- or fifteen-minute walk at a relatively leisurely pace. After several days, you can begin to increase walking time. Then you can increase the pace as well as the length of the walk. It makes good sense to spend a month or even more at building up your walking stamina without adding any other activity.

Basic Principles. There are certain key principles to be followed to gain the most from physical activity.

One is tolerance. You should make no sudden demand on your body for a burst of effort. Excessive straining accomplishes nothing and may lead to injury.

A second principle is overload. After you have become accustomed to exercise, push a little. Easy workouts continued endlessly day after day have only limited value. So start easily and then gradually begin to work a bit harder. Where at first you worked only as long as you felt comfortable, now work just a bit beyond the first feeling of tiredness—just a bit, not to excess. Remember, your heart and body have more capacity than they are usually called upon to use. Give them a little more load than usual and they can handle it. Progressively, they will become able to handle more.

Progression is another key principle. As you continue with a regular schedule of activity and as your strength and endurance increase, your activities will become easier for you. If you continue them at the same level, you will maintain improvement. To go beyond, you can make the workouts progressively more strenuous—if your physician allows—until you arrive at a fitness level you want to achieve.

A Balanced Program. Most people understand how specific exercises for specific muscles can increase their strength and size. If you consider bulging arm biceps desirable, fine. But don't concentrate exclusively on exercises for the biceps. Tone up other muscles—including those of the abdominal area and the back.

If a program is to be balanced, it should train the heart and generally improve the circulation, too. And the best activities for these purposes are those that are continuous—such as brisk walking, jogging, swimming.

There is no best way to build up fitness. One way, as we have suggested, is to start with walking and continue that for a month or more. You can then begin to intersperse jogging with the walking, starting perhaps with fifty steps of jogging, then walking four or five minutes, then jogging another fifty steps and so on. Gradually, you can jog for longer periods.

Running in place indoors is also of value. Begin this, too, gradually. Count as one step each time your left foot touches the floor. For the first few days, run 100 steps at a pace of 100 or fewer steps per minute. Gradually work up to 1,500 steps or more. Fifteen minutes of this a day, kept up regularly every day, can build endurance.

You can then add sit-ups and push-ups and other exercises.

If you would like additional suggestions for a home exercise program, you can write for the following publications:

Adult Physical Fitness. President's Council on Physical Fitness. Superintendent of Documents, U.S. Government Printing Office, Washington, D.C. 20402.

Physical Fitness. Department of Health Education, American Medical Association, 535 North Dearborn, Chicago, Illinois 60610.

Seven Paths to Fitness. From the same source.

Does an exercise program take too much time? Not really. Fifteen to thirty minutes a day is not an inordinate amount of time. Many of us spend several hours a day eating and drinking to less advantage, if not to outright disadvantage. Why not invest some of this time in exercise?

Thus, the outlook today from the standpoint of prevention is increasingly promising.

There is growing evidence that we are gaining valuable insights into atherosclerosis and how it develops and progresses to produce coronary heart disease. No longer is the disease regarded, as it was just a few decades ago, as something inevitable with aging. We know it *is* a disease to be fought, not something to be accepted as inevitable.

Undoubtedly we have much more to learn about it, but it seems almost certain that we can make marked inroads on the disease, that we can significantly reduce our risks, by using diet (and when necessary drugs) to reduce elevated levels of cholesterol and triglycerides, by exercising regularly, by avoiding cigarette smoking, by controlling high blood pressure, diabetes, gout and other disorders that favor atherosclerosis and by reducing emotional stresses as much as possible.

[15]

Drugs for the Heart

Many drugs affect the heart and circulation. A few are old; many are new. In this chapter, we will discuss the key "cardiac drugs" which play the major part in treatment of heart disease.

We think, as do most physicians, that it is important for patients to have a basic understanding of drugs that may be prescribed for them. For generally drugs which are effective are potent. It is their potency that makes them effective, but because they are potent, they can cause trouble if misused. An informed patient can participate most helpfully in his own treatment.

DIGITALIS AND RELATED PREPARATIONS

Digitalis is the most widely used drug in the treatment of many cardiac conditions, including abnormal rhythms and heart failure. There are patients taking it on a long-term basis in all parts of the world.

194

Digitalis has two principal properties which make it valuable:

1. It has a tonic effect on the heart. It helps the heart to pump out more blood with each contraction. It appears to help the heart muscle make better use of energy and thus increase its efficiency. As a result, digitalis is valuable in cases of congestive heart failure. As the failing heart is strengthened and becomes able to pump more blood, congestion in the lungs, the liver and the legs may disappear.

2. Digitalis has a delaying effect on impulses from the atria to the ventricles, making it valuable when too many impulses cause the ventricles to contract excessively and inefficiently. Digitalis is capable of slowing down the ventricular rate to a desired level, which often results in dramatic improvement of the patient's condition.

Some patients believe that if digitalis is prescribed, they must be suffering from irreversible damage to the heart. This is not necessarily the case at all. As we noted, digitalis is used to break the vicious cycle of heart failure; treatment with it can eliminate as much as 20 pounds of excess fluid from the body and return a heart which has failed to its essentially normal function, thereby allowing a patient to live many productive years without significant limitation on activities.

Digitalis may also be used for a patient who has only a rapid heart rate without any organic disease. And it may be used on a prophylactic or preventive basis for patients with heart disease who are about to undergo stressful situations such as surgery or childbirth, to strengthen their hearts so that heart failure will not develop.

Many preparations of digitalis are now available. They include digitalis folia (leaf), digoxin, digitoxin, gitalin, lanatoside C, ouabain and strophanthin. Some are more rapid-acting than others; some, longer-lasting. Some can be given by injection; others can be taken by mouth. The physician can choose from them, depending on the particular needs of the patient.

But digitalis preparations cannot be taken indiscriminately. Excessive amounts can have a poisonous effect on the heart muscle. Digitalis is usually given two or three times a day for a few days—

this is called the digitalizing dose—and then continued once a day in what is called a maintenance dose.

Patients vary in their sensitivity to the drug, and a proper dose for the individual patient must be established and maintained. Among the undesirable but not serious reactions to excessive doses are loss of appetite, nausea, vomiting, and diarrhea. These symptoms provide a convenient warning that the dose is too high, and the patient should report them so the dose can be properly adjusted.

Among the potentially serious reactions to excessive digitalis are abnormal heart rhythms. The drug in excess can produce nearly all the known rhythm disturbances. When it does, it may have to be stopped immediately until the disturbance is eliminated, then started again at a more suitable time.

There is some evidence that patients who have lost large amounts of potassium from the body are prone to develop symptoms of digitalis excess. Certain drugs may produce this potassium loss. They include diuretics, cortisone and cathartics. Such potassium loss can be compensated for through the use of fresh orange juice, cranberry juice and any broth with high potassium content.

DIURETICS

These are drugs which eliminate excess fluid from the body, with particular effectiveness against fluid accumulated as a result of heart failure. The introduction of modern diuretics has revolutionized treatment of heart failure by virtually eliminating once-dreaded "dropsy." While digitalis is used to improve the function of the failing heart directly, diuretic treatment may be added to relieve the consequences of the heart failure and in so doing reduce the load on the heart.

Early diuretic agents included derivatives of caffeine (coffee and tea are weak diuretics). Among the most important currently used diuretics are (1) organic compounds of mercury such as meralluride and mercaptomerin, which are most effective when given by injection; (2) drugs of the thiazide family, which include chlorothiazide, hydroclorothiazide, trichlormethiazide, benzoflumethiazide, polythiazide, benzthiazide, and hydroflumethiazide—all of which may be taken by mouth; (3) drugs of the phthalimidine family, which includes chlorthalidone—all taken by mouth. There are others as well, including spironolactone, theophylline and ethacrynic acid.

Diuretics act on the kidneys to increase elimination of sodium and water from the blood, which in turn is replaced from the waterlogged tissues of the patient. If a patient has severe heart failure and must get rid of fluids quickly, a potent diuretic given by injection can, within just five to ten minutes, produce a marked increase in urine flow, leading to quick relief of shortness of breath caused by lung congestion. Some of the drugs taken by mouth are effective within an hour or two and may remain effective for twelve to twenty-four hours.

The diuretics are extremely valuable, but, like virtually all valuable drugs, they may have undesirable effects on occasion. After long use they may lead to loss of excessive amounts of potassium, which may cause muscle weakness, decreased bowel function and a feeling of prostration. If a patient is on digitalis, the potassium loss may lead to symptoms of excess digitalis. Sometimes the use of orange juice will supply enough potassium to compensate; if not, other potassium supplements can be used.

Sometimes prolonged diuretic treatment will increase the level of uric acid in the blood and lead to gout. When this occurs, the drug may have to be withdrawn, or standard effective treatment for the gout may be used.

Rarely, a patient has some particular sensitivity to a diuretic agent which may lead to jaundice or a skin rash. When this occurs, another diuretic may be substituted.

ANTIARRHYTHMIC DRUGS

These are lifesaving drugs. They combat many types of abnormal heart rhythms, including the very serious. As we have noted, many people have died of heart attacks although their hearts were really too good to die. They were victims of abnormal rhythms. The use of modern antiarrhythmic drugs in coronary care units today is restoring many thousands of patients each year to normal or near-normal living. Never before have so many of these drugs been available.

We have already mentioned digitalis as being an antiarrhythmic agent as well as a tonic for the heart. Now, let's look at the other lifesaving drugs.

Quinidine, derived from the bark of the tropical cinchona tree and related to quinine, is an effective antiarrhythmic drug. Its principal effect is to reduce or eliminate excessive impulses within the heart which can lead to premature beats and episodes of rapid heart action. Quinidine acts quickly and for short periods of time; therefore, it has to be administered several times a day. In addition to stopping abnormal rhythms, it can be used to prevent recurrences.

In some patients, quinidine produces such side effects as ringing of the ears, dizziness, visual disturbances, headache, nausea, vomiting, diarrhea, fever, skin eruption. When these occur, it may be necessary to stop the drug or reduce the dosage.

Procaine amide is a drug originally used as a local anesthetic. It is a derivative of the well-known Novocain. It is useful in eliminating some abnormal heart actions, and is similar in action to quinidine. It may produce side effects in the form of skin eruptions or gastrointestinal complaints.

Lidocaine is a valuable drug for stopping ventricular tachycardia (very rapid beating of the heart). It is used especially in people who develop undesirable reactions to quinidine or procaine amide. It is given by injection into a vein.

Dilantin, a drug often used in the treatment of epilepsy, is also valuable in the treatment of abnormal rhythms.

Propranolol is a new drug, one of a group of beta adrenergic blocking agents from which other valuable antiarrhythmic drugs may be developed. Given by injection or by mouth, it tends to reduce the excitability of the heart muscle and its rate of contraction. Its side effects may include lightheadedness, drowsiness, flushing, confusion.

Isoproterenol is a valuable drug for patients who have slowing of the heartbeat, for it increases the heart rate and also has beneficial effects on the force of the heart contraction.

ANTIANGINAL DRUGS

As we have seen, nitroglycerin is valuable for the relief of chest pain caused by inadequate blood supply to the heart (angina pectoris). It seems to work by dilating the coronary arteries, thus allowing more blood to reach the heart muscle. It also apparently reduces the work load on the heart by dilating arteries elsewhere in the body. In any case, it is a drug that works, and works well. It is most effective when placed under the tongue, where it is dissolved by saliva and rapidly absorbed, producing almost instantaneous relief.

Nitroglycerin is not only rapid-acting but short-acting. Its major purpose is to end an attack of pain when it occurs or to prevent an attack under circumstances conducive to one. Once the action of the drug is completed, usually in a matter of minutes, it has no further effect. When it is needed, therefore, nitroglycerin may be taken many times a day.

There are other drugs, called nitrates, which are related to nitroglycerin. They appear to act similarly but have longer-lasting effects.

ANTICOAGULANTS

In the 1920's, herds of cattle developed hemorrhages and bled to death after eating rotted sweet clover hay. The affliction came to be known as "sweet clover disease." Then, in 1933, a farmer who had lost five cows because of the disease took the carcass of one to the University of Wisconsin in an effort to determine why clover made the cow bleed to death.

Dr. Karl Link, an agricultural chemist, removed some of the animal's blood and tried to make it clot in a test tube but it wouldn't. For the next six years, Link and his associates studied rotted sweet clover and finally found in it a substance called dicoumarin. Coumarin is a chemical which gives sweet clover its aroma; it turns into dicoumarin when hay rots. In animal tests, the scientists found that they could make blood become more fluid with dicoumarin. In 1941, a new drug called dicumarol was used on human patients to prevent blood clotting and vein inflammation after surgery. Soon, other anticoagulant, or anticlotting, drugs became available.

Anticoagulant drugs may be used in heart patients when it is considered necessary to overcome any tendency to clotting within the heart and blood vessels.

There are two types of anticoagulants. One acts directly on the clotting mechanism by interfering with the chain of chemical events leading to blood clotting. This type is represented by *heparin*, a powerful substance normally present in the body. The other type, which includes a variety of chemicals related to coumarin, acts primarily on the liver and prevents the formation there of prothrombin, one of the substances needed for clotting.

Heparin, which is injected, has a short-lived effect and must be administered several times a day. It is usually considered most suitable for short-term treatment. Coumarin derivatives and other similarly acting synthetic drugs act more slowly and are effective when taken in tablet form; they are usually employed for long-term treatment.

When anticoagulants are used, their effects must be carefully evaluated if clotting is to be prevented without risk of internal hemorrhage or excessive bleeding from minor cuts. Therefore, periodic tests are made. With heparin, a direct measurement of clotting time in a sample of the patient's blood provides an indication of efficacy. When the other type of anticoagulants is used, a prothrombin test is made to ensure that prothrombin is not reduced enough for hemorrhaging to occur.

ANTILIPIDEMIC DRUGS

These are drugs which can reduce the level of cholesterol and other lipids, or fatty substances, in the blood.

In most patients who have abnormally high lipid levels which may increase their risk of developing coronary-artery disease, diet, as we have seen in Chapter 14, constitutes prime treatment. The vast majority respond to weight reduction and a diet that is low in saturated fat and cholesterol. For those patients not sufficiently benefited by diet, drug treatment may be added:

Clofibrate is one of the most useful of the lipid-lowering drugs. It both interferes with the body's manufacture of cholesterol and increases cholesterol excretion. It also reduces abnormally high levels of triglycerides (the most common fatty substances in the blood), although how it does this is unknown.

Most patients tolerate clofibrate well, but there are occasional adverse reactions, such as nausea, skin outbreaks and sore muscles. Clofibrate interacts with oral anticoagulants, and if such an anticoagulant is being used, the dose must usually be reduced by a third to a half to prevent bleeding.

Sodium dextrothyroxine is often effective in lowering cholesterol, although the mechanism of its action is not known. The proper dose must be carefully determined so that the individual patient can avoid side effects such as nervousness and diarrhea. In some patients, it may cause angina.

Nicotinic acid also lowers cholesterol, but its side effects are more pronounced than those of the two preceding drugs. Side effects include skin flushing, itching, gastrointestinal upsets, elevation of blood sugar and uric acid and sometimes liver-function abnormality. The appearance and degree of side effects are related to the dose of nicotinic acid. But in some patients, it is possible to find a dose which produces minimal or no discomfort and is effective in lowering cholesterol and triglyceride levels.

Sitosterols, if taken before meals, interfere with the absorption of cholesterol from food and bile. They tend to lower cholesterol.

When necessary, the physician may prescribe combinations of two or more of the preceding drugs to achieve better results with minimal side effects.

OTHER DRUGS

The physician has available many other drugs for use in the treatment of diseases of the heart and circulation.

Antihypertensive drugs, which reduce elevated blood-pressure levels, are often of great importance. These have been discussed in some detail in Chapter 6.

Antibiotics play an important part in the treatment of rheumatic fever and heart infections. Penicillin is commonly used and highly effective. In some instances, because of the nature of a particular organism involved in a heart infection, the physician may choose an antibiotic which may be specifically effective against that organism. The list of available antibiotics is a long one.

Sedatives and tranquilizers are sometimes valuable for controlling restlessness, anxiety and other disturbing symptoms.

Pain-killers and sleeping tablets are frequently needed and serve very useful purposes for patients with heart problems.

[16]

Surgery to Revitalize the Heart

Not long ago, after a series of heart attacks, a fifty-year-old man was wheeled into an operating room. For the next nine hours surgeons worked to rehabilitate his seemingly doomed heart. They cut away an abnormally ballooned-out, weakened section the size of an orange, then stitched together the remaining relatively healthy heart muscle.

They removed a vein from a leg, cut it in two and grafted the two sections so they could bypass blood around severely obstructed areas in two coronary arteries. As another means of getting more circulation to his starved heart, they implanted an artery taken from behind the chest wall into a tunnel they made in the heart muscle.

Today the man is back at full-time work as a school guidance counselor. Unable before to take even a few steps without agonizing chest pain, he now keeps himself in trim with a daily exercise routine of jogging, push-ups and sit-ups.

He is one of a growing number of beneficiaries of an aggressive use of surgery as a means of combating coronary heart disease. There were many attempts in the past to renew the supply of blood for the heart muscle when it had been seriously impaired by disease. Most had to be abandoned, because they produced no clear benefits and carried high risk of death on the operating table.

Today, however, there are several types of surgical procedures which appear to be capable of improving function and extending life when medical measures have failed.

HELP FROM A CHEST ARTERY

Modern surgical efforts to revascularize the heart muscle—provide it with new blood supply—go back to 1945, when Dr. Arthur Vineberg of the Royal Victoria Hospital, Montreal, thought of using the internal mammary artery as a new channel for the ailing heart.

The artery runs down behind the chest wall, supplying certain chest areas with blood. Because other arteries also supply these areas, the internal mammary could be spared. Dr. Vineberg had the idea that the artery could be freed from its attachments to the chest wall, brought over to the heart muscle, and placed in a little tunnel made in the heart muscle. The hope was that when so implanted, the artery might give rise to small collateral blood vessels which would become hooked up with unblocked branch coronary arteries, thus establishing a new network for circulation.

Vineberg spent many years in experimental work with animals before trying the procedure in human patients. After he had used it in 150 patients—all of whom had serious heart trouble and two-thirds of whom had suffered at least one heart attack—he reported that about 70 percent appeared to have benefited. They felt better, could be more active.

While there was interest in Vineberg's work, there was need for clear objective proof that a transplanted mammary artery actually remains open and does not shrivel up and become useless after a time. Finally, in 1962, at the Cleveland Clinic, Dr. F. Mason Sones, Jr., using the then-new technique of cine arteriography (see page 24), studied one of Dr. Vineberg's patients.

The patient had undergone the operation six years before. The artery, the special X-ray studies indicated, was still functioning and collateral circulation had been established.

Technical refinements and additions to the procedure have been made by many surgeons and by Dr. Vineberg himself.

In some patients, so much of the coronary artery system is affected by disease that no single artery implant is likely to be enough to reestablish adequate blood supply. So in November, 1962, Dr. Vineberg began to use a three-step operation. He transplanted the internal mammary artery; stripped away the epicardium, the inner layer of the sac that encloses the heart, to encourage growth of new branches in the coronary network; and grafted a section of the omentum, a blood-rich apron surrounding the abdominal organs, to the heart muscle, so that the omentum would shoot out new blood vessels into the heart muscle.

While the transplant procedure and its variations have helped some patients, it has a drawback in the time lag. Renewed blood flow to the heart muscle is achieved slowly. It may take as long as six months after surgery before new circulation pathways are established. Until this happens, the patient does not benefit, and he may not be able to survive that long.

OPERATING ON BLOCKED ARTERIES

Hoping for quicker results, surgeons began a direct attack on blocked coronary arteries. In one procedure called endarterotomy, fatty deposits clogging a local area of coronary artery are left intact, but the artery wall in the area is slit open and a patch of vein or other material is sewn to the wall. In this way the caliber, or bore, of the vessel is enlarged so that more blood can pass through.

Another procedure approaches the same problem in a different way. When a section of artery is blocked, the artery is opened, the obstructing material is surgically stripped away with a circular knife to widen the channel, then the artery is closed again. The procedure is called endarterectomy.

A newer version of endarterectomy makes use of gas rather than a knife. A jet of carbon dioxide is injected into a blocked vessel. The high-pressure jet of gas separates the obstructing material from the artery, so the material can be removed. Gas endarterectomy takes less time. It has been used with some success to overcome obstructions in blood vessels of the neck, abdomen and legs. There is some hope that the procedure may be more effective in coronary heart disease than conventional endarterectomy is; for while the knife frees the core of a main coronary artery, it cannot remove obstructions in side branches of the artery. With gas, however, the surgeon can follow the contours of arterial walls and loosen obstructions in side branches as well.

Both endarterotomy and endarterectomy are suitable for only a limited number of patients—those with small lengths of artery clogged by deposits.

BYPASSING THE BLOCKS

When an artery is blocked elsewhere in the body, such as in a leg, it has sometimes been possible to provide for a detour that takes blood around the block. Now bypassing has become a promising means of treating blocks in the coronary circulation. In recent years advances in this field have been quite rapid.

One method of bypassing connects the internal mammary artery directly to a coronary artery beyond the diseased area. Blood then flows from the internal mammary into the healthy section of coronary artery and on to feed the heart muscle.

Another method is to use a saphenous vein taken from the patient's leg. The saphenous vein is a large vessel running the length of each leg. It returns about 10 percent of the blood in the leg to the heart. But it can be spared, for other veins can take over its work. And, in fact, this is the vein which is commonly removed in varicose-vein surgery.

For a vein bypass, one end of the vein is inserted into the aorta, the body's main trunkline. The other end is inserted into a coronary artery beyond the point of obstruction.

Much of the pioneering work in vein bypassing for coronary

heart disease has been done by Dr. René G. Favaloro at the Cleveland Clinic and Dr. W. Dudley Johnson of Marquette University and St. Luke's Hospital, Milwaukee. Begun only as recently as 1967, the work has proceeded rapidly.

You will recall that two main coronary arteries—a right and a left—come off the aorta. The right runs a moderately long course down the front of the heart before dividing into two branches, one of which continues down while the other goes around to the back of the heart. The left coronary runs a short course and also divides into a branch which supplies the front part of the heart, and another which goes around to the back.

In their vein-grafting work at first, surgeons were able to bypass blocks only high up in the right coronary artery, because it is a relatively easy area to reach. The artery diameter is larger here, and stitching a vein to it is a less formidable task. But while such bypasses may help 5 to 10 percent of patients, others have obstructions lower down and often in both left and right coronary arteries.

An emergency situation helped to extend the usefulness of vein grafting. One morning in July, 1968, Dr. Johnson was operating on a patient with an aneurysm, a ballooned-out section of the front of the left ventricle. He had removed the aneurysm when suddenly the diseased right coronary artery closed off at a point around in back of the heart. With its back wall no longer receiving blood because of the closed-off artery, the ventricle could not contract. The patient had been placed on a heart-lung machine for the aneurysm operation. He was still on the machine but it can be used for only a few hours; after that, it may produce deadly damage.

Unless, somehow, the ventricle could be made to contract again, the patient had no chance to live. There was only one hope: a long vein graft from the aorta to a clear, unblocked portion of the small right coronary artery branch in back of the heart. The graft worked; with its circulation restored, the ventricle started contracting again.

The immediate success, of course, was gratifying. And the operation opened up broader possibilities. A vein had been attached to a tiny coronary branch only 1½ millimeters in diameter. If that could be done in back of the heart, it should be possible in front of the heart. If an artery had a major obstruction high up and also had smaller blocks lower down, it should be possible to go beyond the last diseased segment and graft to a healthy vessel where the diameter might be as small as 1½ millimeters. And perhaps that could be done in the left as well as the right coronary artery.

Dr. Johnson was soon able to report success in such grafting in patients with right coronary artery disease and then in others with left coronary artery disease. Late in 1968, he was able to go a step further and do a double bypass. Within a year after that, ninety patients at the Milwaukee hospital had been given double and triple vein bypasses—two and three lengths of saphenous vein attached at the aorta and running to clear portions of right coronary and to both branches of the left coronary.

Currently, more than fifty surgical groups across the country are aggressively exploring the values of surgery for patients with coronary heart disease who are beyond help in other ways. Often, they combine several techniques to fit the needs of the individual patient. They use bypass vein grafts, internal mammary implants, gas endarterectomy. When necessary, they remove aneurysms at the same time.

HOW AN OPERATION GOES

Typically, before a patient is considered a possible candidate for surgery, X-ray movies of the coronary arteries are taken to reveal what goes on inside the arteries and where there are points of obstruction. When the patient arrives in the operating room, there is a well-defined plan of approach.

The surgeon is assisted by a sizable and well-trained team, including assisting surgeons, anesthesiologists, two or more nurses, a heart-lung-machine technician and a technician for the electronic equipment that keeps monitoring the patient all through surgery.

The operation starts with an incision in a leg to remove a long segment of saphenous vein from groin to knee. At the same time, the patient's chest is being opened. After the vein is removed, it is thoroughly tested. One end is pinched, a syringe is inserted into the other end, and the vein is inflated with saline solution. Any tiny leaks are sewn up.

Now the patient is connected to the heart-lung machine, which takes over the work of pumping blood and adding oxygen to it and removing carbon dioxide. If there is an aneurysm, this useless ballooned-out portion of the heart is removed and the remainder is stitched together.

The surgeon briefly touches two electrodes to the heart. Instantly, the heart begins to fibrillate, quivering rather than contracting forcefully. This provides a quieter field in which the surgeon can work. Tissue overlying the coronary arteries is cut away, and it becomes possible to see the yellowish atherosclerotic deposits right through the artery walls. Healthy areas of arteries are selected to receive the vein grafts.

A clamp is placed on the aorta to shut off blood flow to the coronary arteries. This causes the heart to stop beating completely, but that is all right because during standstill the heart needs very little nourishment. Furthermore, the clamp is released periodically so blood can flow to provide the necessary nourishment.

The surgeon, working during the standstill periods, makes a tiny slit in an artery and stitches one end of a vein segment to the artery, using suture material as fine as hair. The other end of the vein is stitched to a slit in the aorta. The procedure is repeated for the other bypasses.

With the bypasses completed, the patient can be disconnected from the heart-lung machine. Often improvement is immediately obvious. The heart muscle is getting more blood through the bypasses. The ventricle, freed of the aneurysm that previously acted as a drag on its performance, is working vigorously.

The operation is long. From the beginning to the point where the aneurysm is removed may take ninety minutes. Each vein graft may require an hour. And then, in some patients, another ninety-minute procedure may begin: dissecting out the mammary artery from behind the chest wall and implanting it into the heart wall.

When, at last, the patient's chest is closed and he is ready to be taken from operating room to recovery room, the total procedure may have required eight or nine hours.

To bring a patient with severe coronary heart disease through such an operation has required development of advanced techniques. Before surgery starts, a medication such as digitalis may be used to strengthen the heart. Transfusions may be used before operation if blood volume is low.

As often as every fifteen minutes throughout surgery, by means of instrumentation applied before the operation starts, checks are made on blood levels of oxygen and carbon dioxide, the blood's acid-alkaline balance and other factors. At the slightest indication of a disturbance in any important factor, corrective measures are immediately instituted.

Afterward, in the intensive-care unit where the patient spends the next several days, similar monitoring is carried out repeatedly and corrective measures are used as needed to prevent trouble.

RESULTS

Surgery for coronary heart disease is long, complex and trying. Patients selected for it have been the seriously ill who have not responded to other measures. At one institution, for example, 68 percent of patients operated on had had one to six heart attacks; 52 percent had severe disease of all three coronary arteries; and 16 percent were aged sixty to seventy-two.

At that institution, the mortality rate in the first several hundred operations ran about 14 percent With further refinements in techniques, it has been reduced to 7 percent. That is still higher than anyone would like it to be, but it may well come down even more. And there may be further reduction in mortality as the result not only of further improvement in operative technique, but also as the result of earlier operation.

In the beginning years of any major operative technique, when it must still be regarded as experimental, its application is usually limited to very severe cases. Later, with definitive proof of efficacy, the technique may be used for patients in earlier stages of disease, when chances for success are likely to be greater.

The big question, which only time can answer, is how durable the results are. The immediate benefits are often dramatic. Patients may be freed of incapacitating angina. They may be able to return to virtually normal living, including jobs.

Will these benefits last? Will the newly established circulatory routes remain open and functioning? Thus far, based on repeat X-ray movie studies after a year and eighteen months, the outlook seems promising.

Surgery for coronary heart disease can never be curative. At best, it can rehabilitate, provide a kind of second chance. It does not remove the underlying disease process; it only compensates for the manifestations of the disease process. It would be better if preventive methods could be used to avoid or so retard atherosclerosis that surgery would be unnecessary. And even when surgery is employed, it is still important to apply preventive techniques in the hope that recurrence may be avoided.

Surgery is far from being a routine measure and very probably never will be one. Not every patient with coronary heart disease needs surgery; not every patient can expect to benefit. But surgery gives every indication of being able to make a significant contribution to extending life and enabling it to be more productive and enjoyable for many victims of coronary heart disease.

[17]

Biomedical Engineering
and the Heart

The human body is a marvelously precise and complex machine. Today, as medical researchers study methods to repair the body's machinery, they are finding it rewarding to work closely with engineers, men whose basic concern is the study of machines. A whole new field of specialization in modern medicine, called bioengineering, has been developing. It can be defined as the application of the concepts and methods of engineering and the physical sciences to problems in medicine and biology. Physicists working in this field are referred to as medical physicists.

Among the tremendously valuable early contributions of bioengineers and medical physicists have been the electrocardiograph and the heart-lung machine. Their work has led to the small electronic heart pacers now used by thousands of patients whose hearts must be stimulated to keep beating smoothly.

Both the coronary care unit in the hospital and the more recently developed mobile coronary care unit that goes out from the hospital to the patient are bioengineering contributions. And we appear to be on the threshold of other major bioengineering breakthroughs for patients with heart problems.

CORONARY CARE UNITS

Along a hospital corridor several small rooms are set off by glass partitions and green curtains. Within the rooms, heart-attack patients, pale and quiet, lie in their beds. Some are being attended by doctors or nurses. In the corridor, other doctors and nurses work over charts.

Suddenly, a high-pitched tone, insistent though not loud, breaks the quiet. Everyone looks up at once. The tone signals an emergency. Near one patient's bed, a sweep hand has begun to move on a wall clock and an automatic pen has started to trace a squiggly line across a roll of graph paper.

This is a coronary care unit (CCU). It consists of special equipment and a special hospital team concerned with preventing many crises for heart-attack patients and with reacting instantly to save life when a crisis does occur.

In a typical CCU, every beat of a patient's heart is monitored automatically. Whenever the number of beats drops below 50 a minute or rises above 150, the alarm goes off, the clock starts and an electrocardiograph machine begins to trace the line that records in detail the kind of beats the injured heart is producing. Nurses and physicians can tell immediately not only which patient is in trouble but also, from the clock, when the trouble began and usually, from the electrocardiogram, what is wrong.

As we have said, a heart damaged by a heart attack is made irritable by the damage, particularly in the first hours and days after the attack. Abnormal rhythms may develop, and the heart may even go into a condition called ventricular fibrillation—a state of disorganized, unproductive beating in which the heart, as surgeons sometimes put it, looks and feels like a bag of writhing worms. Or the heart may suddenly stop beating, a situation called sudden cardiac arrest.

A heart beating abnormally or even completely stopped can often be returned to normal beating if the right kind of treatment is immediately available. In a CCU, it *is* immediately available.

Many years ago, Dr. Claude Beck of Cleveland coined a phrase, "hearts too good to die." He was trying to emphasize the merits of making every possible effort to revive victims of sudden heart stoppage. Very often, he noted, their hearts were still essentially sound. They were the victims not of too much basic damage to the heart muscle but of irritability of the muscle during the early hours and days after a heart attack. If they could be revived, he felt, they might well live many years and even normal lifetimes.

CCU's have proved that Dr. Beck was right. Moreover, they have shown that in addition to reviving patients after heart standstill, the CCU approach, with its monitoring equipment and prompt treatment, can often prevent fibrillation from progressing to heart standstill and can even stop other, less serious abnormal rhythms from progressing to fibrillation.

Among the most frequent rhythm abnormalities for heart-attack patients is ventricular extrasystole, or premature contraction. When this is signaled through the CCU monitoring equipment, antiarrhythmic medication can be given at once to suppress the premature contraction and avoid the possibility of more dangerous rhythm abnormality. Often premature contraction disappears within a few days, and the medication can then be tapered off.

One of the more serious arrhythmias is ventricular tachycardia —exceedingly rapid heart action, reaching as many as 250 beats per minute. Often drugs can stop it. When drugs do not work, cardioversion can be used: a quick, intense electrical shock delivered through the chest wall and timed for delivery at a precise instant in the heart cycle.

One physician used a sports picture to describe cardioversion. Imagine, he said, an eight-oared racing shell. One crew member is off stroke. The coxswain's trick is to stop all crew members momentarily until the stroke can be made uniform again.

Cardioversion stops an abnormally beating heart; when, almost instantly, the heart starts beating again, the rhythm is normal.

Another rhythm abnormality, atrial fibrillation—irregular convulsive movements of the upper chambers of the heart—often yields to prompt treatment with drugs or can be terminated by cardioversion.

Bradycardia—abnormally slow heart action—is another frequent problem. An episode or two may be of little consequence. But sustained bradycardia, which can lead to serious difficulties, yields to drug treatment.

CCU's represent a tremendous advance in the treatment of heart-attack patients. They have halved the death rate among hospitalized heart-attack victims.

MOBILE CORONARY CARE UNITS

While CCU's in hospitals are saving many thousands of lives, they can do nothing for patients who do not reach the hospital alive after a heart attack, and as many as two-thirds of all heart-attack deaths occur outside the hospital.

Many of these early deaths stem from heart rhythm derangements. Ventricular fibrillation, deadly unless overcome within about a minute, most often occurs immediately after a heart attack and is less and less likely to develop as time passes.

It is obviously necessary, if the death rate is to be reduced, to make available suitable medical aid without delay. One approach is to equip and staff special ambulances as coronary care units on wheels.

The mobile CCU concept was developed by Dr. J. F. Pantridge and Dr. J. S. Geddes of the Royal Victoria Hospital in Belfast, Ireland. In the first two years, even as it was being tested and refined, the Belfast mobile dashed to the aid of 550 heart-attack victims. By shocking their hearts back into normal rhythm, by administering drugs and fluids and by giving cardiac massage, the mobile staff saved a large number of these patients.

Similar mobile CCU's have gone into use in several cities in Britain. Russia also has a number. Now we in the United States are beginning to have them. Among the first in this country is the one operated by St. Vincent's Hospital in New York City. It responds when a victim or his family calls or when an onlooker dials 911, the city's emergency telephone number.

Mobile CCU's, both here and abroad, have established that a medical team can be mobilized and delivered outside a hospital and that heart-attack victims can be treated on the spot and often saved.

Unfortunately, many hospitals lack the house physician staff to man mobile coronary care units. But there is hope that this problem can be solved by using specially trained nurses and technicians and by allocating enough emergency radio bands for medical use. Given such bands, electrocardiograms could be transmitted from the mobile CCU back to the hospital for quick interpretation by a physician, and nurses and technicians could then act on a physician's instructions.

There is the further problem of educating the patient: if a mobile CCU is to achieve its full lifesaving potential, it must be called for without delay. And so it is necessary to educate people to reach for the phone instead of an antacid when they experience chest pain.

PACEMAKERS

Electronic pacemakers today are keeping the hearts of thousands of people beating despite chronic cardiac disease. And they have revolutionized the treatment of heart block.

Normally the heart is paced by electrical impulses which originate in a collection of cells, called the sino-atrial node, in the upper right quarter of the right atrium. The impulses travel through muscle fibers to initiate contraction of both atria. They also activate another bundle of cells, the atrio-ventricular node, in the lower left quarter of the right atrium. From the atrio-ventricular node, the impulses move rapidly to all parts of the left and right ventricles through specialized conduction tissues.

When one or more major elements of the specialized conduction system are disrupted by disease or injury, heart block of varying severity may result. The impulses do not get through properly, and the pumping action of the ventricles is affected. The patient may experience episodes of giddiness, fainting and convulsions as the impaired pumping action leads to diminished blood flow to the brain. Heart block may occur after a heart attack; when it does, it is usually transient. In some other heart conditions, the block may persist.

Fortunately now, when heart block occurs, normal heart rate can be restored and maintained with an artificial pacemaker. Pacemakers are compact electronic devices measuring approximately 2 x 2½ x 1 inches. They are powered by batteries which generally require replacement every two or three years.

One type of pacemaker, called the transthoracic, is placed in position after the chest has been opened by surgery. Its electrodes are anchored in the heart muscle. Its battery unit may be implanted in an under-skin pouch, usually in the abdomen, where it can be reached more readily when replacement is needed.

A second type of pacemaker, the transvenous, is inserted through a vein. A catheter or tube is threaded into the vein and then maneuvered to the heart so the pacemaker electrodes can be introduced through the catheter into the right ventricle.

The first pacemakers operated at a fixed rate. They fired regularly, usually at a rate of about 80 times a minute. Newer, more sophisticated pacemakers now operate on the "demand" principle: They are so designed that they work only when needed. As long as the heart is beating at a desired rate on its own, a demand pacemaker remains out of operation. The instant the heart rate becomes abnormal, the electronic device automatically takes over to restore normal rhythm.

In some patients, artificial pacing may be required for only a short period of time; in others, it may be needed for a prolonged period or even permanently. The physician's choice of a pacemaker is based on the particular needs of an individual patient.

Pacemakers have occasionally failed in the past because of breaks in the wires carrying the pacing pulses to the electrodes. Such failure has required an operation to replace the device. But recently, special wires have been developed to overcome this problem.

Battery failure has not been a frequent cause of pacemaker failure. If a run-down battery has to be replaced, it requires relatively simple surgery to open the skin pouch, remove the battery, insert a new one, and close up the pouch again.

Pacemakers have saved many lives and will save many more. They are constantly being refined to make them more useful. One experimental pacemaker, for example, eliminates the need for wires at all. A transmitter worn outside the body beams radio energy through the chest to a tiny receiver implanted within the sac that encloses the heart. The receiver converts the radio energy to electrical pacing stimuli. Another experimental pacemaker weighs less than one ounce and is powered by a special crystal that changes mechanical energy, derived from ventricular contractions, to electrical energy. A portion of this energy is converted by the crystal to electricity which is stored in a tiny condenser. The stored electricity is then fed as needed to a pulse-generator.

Also being developed is a nuclear-powered pacemaker which scientists hope will run twenty years or more. One current device is about as long as a fingernail and as wide as a cigarette, and is powered by 1/200 of an ounce of plutonium 238. Heat given off by the plutonium is turned into electricity by a thermoelectric converter. Timed bursts of electrical energy conducted to the heart muscle by wires maintain the heartbeat.

There are some who now believe that the development of a reliable long-term pacemaker may make heart transplantation unnecessary. But there is also the possibility that the nuclear power source finally developed for such a pacemaker may one day prove ideal for driving a totally artificial heart.

The results with present-day models are gratifying. For example, one study covered 327 patients who received pacemakers over a ten-year period. At the end of the period, 73 percent remained alive. Of the eighty-seven deaths, many were not related to heart disease. A number of the surviving patients had returned to jobs and virtually normal living.

THE HEART-LUNG MACHINE

Until the heart-lung machine became available, the heart had remained the last frontier for surgery because of the problem of trying to operate on the beating pump without disrupting circulation to vital organs. By introducing a finger into a heart chamber and working blind, the surgeon could provide some degree of relief for a heart-valve obstruction. But more complex heart problems could not be tackled until it became possible to operate, under direct vision, in the open heart, and with time enough to make intricate repairs.

The heart-lung machine, also known as the pump oxygenator, can, as we have seen, take over the pumping work of the heart and the oxygenating work of the lungs, and it can do this for several hours while the surgeon works on the heart.

While there are variations in the way the machine can be used, usually blood returning from the patient's body via the two great veins, the venae cavae, is brought through tubing into the machine. In the artificial-lung part of the device, oxygen is added and carbon dioxide is removed as the blood flows through. This is done by exposing the blood to oxygen or air in large flat disk surfaces, by bubbling oxygen through the blood or by other means. The blood is then pumped into the patient's arterial system. With the heart-lung machine in operation, as we noted in the last chapter, the heart can be opened, its beating stopped and repairs made in a dry and motionless field.

There are at times problems associated with the use of the heart-lung machine. Some patients suffer afterward from psychotic episodes. The reason is not clear. Some investigators believe that the mental problems may develop because tiny blood clots may form in the machine and then lodge in the brain; others, because the pressure produced by the machine is lower than that produced by the normal heart, and the lower pressure may fail to get fully adequate supplies of blood to the brain. Whatever the reason for these psychotic episodes, most patients who develop them recover from them. Generally, the shorter the period of time a patient is on the heart-lung machine, the less the likelihood of complications.

Undoubtedly, there will be improvements in the machine. But even current problems associated with use of the device are vastly overshadowed by the saving of life it has made possible.

And it has been the success with the heart-lung machine—the demonstration that artificial equipment can be used in place of the heart—which has spurred efforts to develop an artificial heart (see Chapter 18).

CINEMATIC MEDICINE

This is a term sometimes applied to a major aid in the battle against heart disease—the X-ray movie technique which allows physicians to see the coronary arteries and what goes on within them.

The technique, which has the formidable technical name of selective cine coronary arteriography, has been discussed earlier (Chapter 2). But it is of such importance that we want to provide additional detail here.

Ordinarily, blood vessels are invisible on X rays and through the fluoroscope, and until this technique was developed major surgery was required for a look at the coronary arteries.

Coronary arteriography works this way. Fully conscious, the patient lies on a table beneath an X-ray machine equipped with a device called an image amplifier. The amplifier brightens X-ray images to permit high-speed motion pictures to be made. Under local anesthesia, a small incision is made in the right arm, an artery is opened, and a thin plastic tube or catheter is inserted into the artery and carefully pushed up until it reaches the aorta. Near this point in the aorta are two small openings leading to the coronary arteries. Carefully, with the aid of the image amplifier, the tip of the catheter is guided into one of the coronary arteries.

A fluid is injected into the catheter, the fluid which will make the vessel visible. The fluid is opaque to X rays and appears black on the screen. As the fluid reaches and fills the coronary artery, a black, treelike image appears on the screen and moves as the heart expands and contracts. In a few seconds, the fluid is washed away and the image disappears. But meanwhile a movie camera has recorded the events on the image screen. The procedure is repeated for the other coronary artery.

It requires about an hour to get a complete view of the coronary arteries. Insertion of the catheter causes little if any discomfort, because the arteries through which it passes have no sensory nerves.

By studying the movies, heart specialists can spot any area where a sudden narrowing of the stream of black fluid indicates an obstruction. They can detect any point where fluid flow suddenly stops because of complete blockage.

It is hardly possible to exaggerate the value of arteriography. It helps evaluate patients in whom the diagnosis of coronary atherosclerosis is not clear-cut. It aids in evaluating patients for whom surgery may be contemplated. It has been helpful in determining the effectiveness of various types of surgery for bypassing or otherwise compensating for coronary-artery narrowing. It is also of value in many cases in demonstrating that what may seem, because of symptoms, to be heart disease is not really heart disease at all (see Chapter 19).

ELECTROCARDIOGRAPHY

The ECG—the chart which depicts the function of the heart's electrical system—is, as you know, a frequently used diagnostic aid. Now a whole series of new developments promises to extend greatly the usefulness of electrocardiography.

For example, it is now possible to use computers to analyze ECG's sent in by telephone from remote clinics. In one experimental program, a central computer at the University of Missouri is serving seven remote stations as far as 300 miles away. The computer receives ECG's, analyzes them and then transmits the results back in plain English.

At Hahnemann Medical College and Hospital in Philadelphia, a new, computerized ECG system, which may serve as a prototype for similar installations in other hospitals, makes it possible for an ECG to be interpreted in about sixty seconds.

Speed is only one of the advantages. Because the computer is programmed with constant criteria, all ECG's can be interpreted consistently, with human variation virtually eliminated. Moreover, the system provides more complete information than has been previously available and the cost per ECG is markedly reduced. Still another advantage is that ECG's can be compared over any given period of time. Because the computer stores the information, it can be presented and analyzed on demand.

The cart used by the technician for the computerized ECG is not much larger than the standard ECG cart. First the technician attaches the leads to the patient. Then, using a dialing card, he calls the computer by phone. The computer verifies the patient identification and signals when it is ready to receive the ECG. When the computer has recorded the information, it signals the technician that it has received the complete message. The computer prints out the ECG chart and the interpretation of the data in about one minute. It takes about five minutes to prepare the patient, communicate with the computer, and record the ECG.

With the new system, not only the twelve leads of a traditional ECG but three additional leads can be programmed. These additional leads show instantaneous electrical events of the heart which have not usually been handled before because it was too time-consuming to interpret their data. Such information was previously taken only on selected patients.

Hahnemann takes and interprets about 100 ECG's daily. The computer can handle 300. Formerly it took five or six doctor-hours a day to read and interpret the ECG's, another hour to check the interpretations. With the new system, it takes only one doctor about a half hour per day to check 100 computer ECG's and interpretations.

With the system, too, it is possible to tie in community hospitals and area nursing homes that have no ECG services of their own.

Many other promising ECG developments are being tested. One produced by the U.S. Public Health Service, is an experimental chair which reduces the time required for taking electrocardiograms. It does away with the need for undressing, for maneuvering on and off a table and for attaching electrodes to the body. The chair itself is wired to the ECG machine and the clothed patient just sits in it, making contact with the electrocardiograph leads in the armrests and footrests. The device may be practical for quick screening of large groups of people.

Another promising device is a pocket-size ECG recorder. Contained in a 3x4½x¾-inch plastic case are a miniature ECG amplifier, tape recorder, heart-rate trigger, alarm and batteries. The alarm can be set to start a recording when a patient's heartbeat reaches a specific upper or lower point—or the patient can trigger the mechanism if he suffers any unexplained pains, dizziness or fullness in his chest.

An example of how the device can be used is the case of a seventeen-year-old girl who had unexplained episodes of rapid heart beat. Periodically, her doctor had treated her with anti-arrhythmic drugs even though he could never find anything wrong on an ECG.

She was shown how to use the device, placing the miniature electrodes over her heart and wearing the tape recorder in a shirt pocket throughout her normal school day. The very next day, during a history test, the girl suffered one of her typical attacks. The recorder revealed a heart beat rate of 150 per minute during the attack. But the ECG showed no abnormal heart function during the attack. With this to go on, physicians could decide that there was nothing seriously wrong with her heart even though the beat increased markedly under the stress of a classroom test and, very likely, under other emotional excitement or stress.

The device promises to provide a simple but powerful diagnostic tool for documenting fleeting abnormal rhythms, and to be a boon for patients with unexplained heart troubles. Hospitalization for testing is expensive. With the little recorder, testing can be done while the patient is in his normal environment. And many times the normal environment may provide important clues that might not be picked up in the hospital.

PRECORONARY CARE

This could be a whole new area of great potential importance, in the view of some bioengineering researchers.

As they see it, coronary care units in hospitals have demonstrated that many lives can be saved when lifesaving measures are instituted without delay once a patient develops a problem. Mobile coronary care units can help save additional lives. But still more is needed.

Actually, experience with coronary care units has shown that very often there are warning minor disorders of heart rhythm before a dangerous life-threatening rhythm disorder develops. The focus in coronary care units accordingly has changed to detecting and treating the less serious disturbances before the grave ones have a chance to develop.

The concept of precoronary care would encourage anyone who has even minor symptoms that might be attributable to the heart to go to a special precoronary care area in a hospital. There, as an outpatient, he could take a seat in a lounge and, while reading or watching television, wear a telemetry unit which would transmit his ECG to a receiver. The receiver would play it into a special device designed to detect indications of abnormal rhythm. If a minor abnormality of rhythm were detected, treatment for it could be started without delay.

Some investigators are convinced that it will be practical to develop pocket-size special monitoring devices to be worn by people who have had heart attacks and by others who have coronary heart disease. The monitoring equipment would instantly alert wearers whenever a potentially dangerous pattern of heart rhythm was detected, thus providing the chance to notify a doctor quickly and get to a hospital in time for lifesaving treatment.

[18]

Heart Transplants and the Artificial Heart

For centuries, man has dreamed of the time when diseased or injured organs of the body could be replaced by healthy ones. Now, after years of intensive research, kidney transplantation has become an accepted treatment for some patients who otherwise would die of kidney disease. Corneas of the eye have been transplanted successfully. And it is expected that before long, transplantation of liver, lung, bone marrow, pancreas, spleen, intestine, bone and other organs and tissues will become reality.

HEART TRANSPLANTS

Late in the afternoon of December 2, 1967, in Cape Town, South Africa, a young girl and her mother were knocked down by an automobile. The mother was killed instantly; the girl suffered severe brain damage. Within five minutes after the accident, she was admitted to Groote Schuur Hospital, where investigation indicated that her brain had been irreversibly damaged. Although she was kept alive artificially, nothing could be done to save her life. In the same hospital, a man was dying of an irreversible heart condition. Permission was granted by the girl's father for her normal heart to be removed and transplanted into the body of the man. The man lived eighteen days.

Within eighteen months after that first human heart transplant, a total of 131 transplants had been performed on 129 people in twenty different countries. There is reason to believe that many more were attempted.

Of the first seventy-two patients to receive transplanted hearts, thirty-two died during the first few months and twenty-two more died before six months were up. Of the next forty-eight patients, twenty-three died in the first month. These seem like grim figures, yet they represent initial mortality for a new procedure performed by fifty-four different surgeons scattered throughout the world.

More recent figures have been little more encouraging. By August, 1971, the total number of heart transplants worldwide had increased to 176, of which 112 were performed in the United States. Twenty-eight of the 173 recipients (three had received two transplants each) were still surviving at this time: ten had lived for three years; six, for two years; five, for a year; and seven for less than a year.

The problem is not with surgical technique.

Well before the first human heart transplant, there had been successful animal heart transplants. In various laboratories, the heart had been removed from a donor dog and, after examination to make certain it was not diseased, placed in a cold saline solution and massaged briefly to fill all the chambers with the cold solution, which would preserve it for thirty to sixty minutes. A heart-lung machine was then attached to the recipient dog to maintain circulation through the body while its heart was removed and the donor heart stitched in its place. After the stitching was completed and the clamps released so blood could start to flow through the sewn-in heart, it began to flutter. Then, one swift electric shock, and it began to beat normally.

After ten years of work and a few months before the first human heart transplant in Cape Town, Dr. Norman E. Shumway of Stanford University could report that he had been able to increase the survival rate in dogs with transplanted hearts up to 75 percent.

Nor were the animals—at Stanford and other investigating centers—heart cripples. Some weeks before the Cape Town operation, Dr. Richard Lower of the Medical College of Virginia showed an impressed medical meeting films of a large brown and white dog running and wagging her tail. Nothing extraordinary about the scene, but the dog was extraordinary: beating in her chest was a heart transplanted from another dog a year before. Not only was she healthy; by the grace of the other dog's heart, she had even borne puppies.

The successes with dogs were encouraging. As a technical procedure, heart transplantation in humans was expected to be simpler. The dog aorta, the main vessel coming out of the heart, is more fragile than the human aorta. Connecting it up to a transplanted heart without damage had presented a challenge; surgeons had met the challenge.

Moreover, Dr. Shumway had recently devised a simplified operative technique. It had been customary in animal work to remove the entire heart from the recipient animal. That meant severing two arteries plus two big veins returning used blood from the rest of the body plus four other major veins carrying back freshly oxygenated blood from the lungs. Then it meant attaching all eight vessels to the transplanted heart.

Dr. Shumway had developed a way to leave about 5 percent of the old heart in place—parts of the walls of the heart chambers to which the six veins are attached. Then the transplanted heart, with just that 5 percent cut away, could be joined to the old heart section, saving much delicate sewing of vessels, cutting operating time in half and increasing safety.

And there had been some important preliminary work with human hearts. Dr. Lower in Virginia had removed hearts from persons dead of massive brain injuries, perfused them with blood, stored them for up to an hour, then got them beating again.

As expected, when the Cape Town operation was performed, there was less trouble than with dogs. The aorta was less of a problem. Dr. Shumway's simplified technique, which Dr. Christiaan Barnard used, worked well.

The big problem, as expected, was rejection: the body's blind stubborn efforts to throw off the potentially lifesaving heart.

If you have ever had a splinter in a finger and seen the finger fester, you've witnessed an example of rejection—of the body's immunological system at work.

That system is essential to protect the body against dangerous invading foes. When infectious agents—bacteria, viruses and others—get into the body, the defense system is alerted by antigens, chemicals produced by the invading organisms. White blood cells (lymphocytes) rush to the site. The lymphocytes produce antibodies, chemicals capable of locking onto and inactivating the organisms.

But, unfortunately for transplant surgeons, that same system operates when a heart or other organ is implanted. The transplanted organ's cells produce antigens, thereby inviting destruction by antibody-producing lymphocytes.

As the lymphocytes converge on it, the implanted organ begins to swell. Eventually, as the lymphocytes infiltrate and overwhelm the donor tissue, the tissue cells die. The patient has a fever and a greatly increased white blood cell count. Soon the graft stops functioning, shrivels, dies. It has been rejected.

Transplantation efforts long had foundered because of the rejection problem. Back in 1920, Dr. Serge Voronoff created something of a sensation when he reported that he had performed testicular grafts from ape to man and between animals. After 162 such operations, he held a press conference in Paris and paraded an aged man, a billy goat and a ram, all supposedly rejuvenated by monkey-gland transplants. While much of the world was impressed, medical authorities were not. For in those days, organs always died after a brief period even when transplanted between individuals of the same species, to say nothing of from monkey to man.

It was not until December, 1954, that Dr. Joseph E. Murray in Boston achieved a successful internal organ transplant: a kidney taken fron one identical twin and implanted in the other. Because they were identical in their genetic make-ups, an organ from one was not regarded by the other's body as a foreign invading agent. The first successful transplant between nonidentical twins came in 1958—and it took two more years before there was a successful transplant between less closely related persons.

To try to prevent rejection, doctors first used massive X-ray doses. But the radiation acted like a biological sledgehammer, killing the tissues that produce the lymphocytes and leaving the patient defenseless against ordinary germs and hence wide open to death from pneumonia or other infection.

Then cortisonelike drugs, such as prednisone, and certain anti-cancer drugs, such as Imuran, were found to help suppress the rejection mechanism. By combining low-dosage radiation with the drugs, surgeons walked a kind of tightrope, trying to keep an organ from being rejected without lowering body defenses so much that the patient died of infection. It was touch-and-go.

Matching for better compatibility between donor and recipient could be a help. Matching began with blood types. Before any blood transfusion, red cells are typed to make certain that compatible blood is used; otherwise, there may be a transfusion reaction, a kind of rejection phenomenon. Blood typing for organ transplantation had only limited value, but it was a step in the right direction.

White cells are used for matching. Drops of serum full of white cells from a potential donor are placed on little disks. The disks contain chemical reagents which can react with certain distinctive antigens on the white cells. The kinds and intensities of the reactions on the disks provide a tissue profile of the donor which can be compared with a profile similarly obtained of the recipient.

Thus, in the first Cape Town operation, the girl whose heart was to be transplanted was found by red-cell typing to have the type O negative blood of a universal donor, meaning there would be no rejection because of blood incompatability. Her white-cell profile was similar enough to the man's to provide hope that his rejection mechanism would not react too strongly against the transplant.

The idea behind matching is that the closer the compatability between donor and recipient, the less drug treatment will be needed to restrain the response which produces rejection and therefore the less likelihood of death from infection.

It didn't work in the first transplant. After eighteen days, the heart was still good but the patient died of pneumonia. For one thing, white-cell analysis was in its very earliest stages; much more remained, and still remains, to be learned about it. Also, the treatment with drugs evidently had been too intense.

Results have since improved. Some heart-transplant recipients have lived for more than eighteen months. But rejection still remains the problem to be overcome, and there are intensive efforts to find more effective solutions.

Many of the measures are highly technical. For example, a preparation called antilymphocyte serum (ALS) is intended to turn the table on the lymphocytes which produce the antibodies that lead to rejection. ALS is made by injecting into horses a lymphocyte-rich extract from thymus glands, spleens and lymph nodes removed from human cadavers. The horses' rejection mechanism produces particles active against the human lymphocytes. Then ALS is extracted from the horses' blood and given to transplant patients with the hope that it will attack their lymphocytes and thus interfere with destruction of the transplants.

Another effort involves lymph draining. The antibody-producing lymphocytes circulate principally in the body's lymphatic system. Through a plastic tube inserted in a lymph duct just above the collarbone, lymphocytes can be drained out by gravity into a plastic bag. As many as 32 billion can be removed daily and separated from the lymph fluid. The fluid can then be returned to the patient.

Still another effort involves the use of small doses of purified antigens to desensitize the patient's defense system so it will not react to a transplanted organ. The principle is similar to that used in antiallergy treatment. For example, a patient with an allergy to ragweed may receive periodic injections of small doses of purified ragweed in an attempt to build up tolerance for natural ragweed.

Human heart transplantation remains an investigative procedure. Undoubtedly, there will be advances in the fight against rejection. The day may well come when heart transplantation can be counted on as a practical procedure. Meanwhile, there is growing optimism that the need for many transplants can be avoided by new techniques for revitalizing the heart through surgical procedures on the coronary arteries (see Chapter 16). And, on the other side, there are the efforts to develop artificial hearts.

THE ARTIFICIAL HEART

Surgeons can replace hopelessly damaged heart valves with artificial valves; they can replace sections of the aorta with plastic vessels. But until very recently, the idea of an implantable artificial heart seemed more fantasy than scientific possibility, and many scientific journals refused to accept research papers describing studies in that direction.

The picture has changed greatly. An artificial heart would essentially be a mechanical device to maintain circulation—a pump. The feasibility in principle of substituting such a mechanical pump for the heart has been demonstrated by the success of the heart-lung machine.

At many institutions now, researchers are at work devising and testing in animals mechanical hearts meant to be implanted in the body and to function for indefinite periods of years. There are many problems to be solved, difficult, but not, it would seem, insurmountable.

One such heart consists of two air-driven pumps made of plastic with flexible rubber bladders which replace the right and left ventricles of the natural heart. The right chamber sends blood to the lungs to receive oxygen; the left pumps oxygenated blood to the body. The device is attached to remnants of the atria of the natural heart. It is also connected to the pulmonary artery and to the aorta. Pumping is achieved by the introduction of air, which causes the bladders to collapse and force blood out. And the beat of the device is triggered by the cluster of pacemaking cells in the remnant of the right atrium of the natural heart. The impulses from the pacemaking cells are amplified by an electronic device which directs contraction of the pumping chambers.

Another artificial heart model, which works on the same principle, has two silicone collapsible ventricles encased in a rigid plastic housing; this device also uses an electronic device to control beating.

These and still other models receive their power supply from consoles outside the body. Before a man can live, breathe and walk with such a device in his chest, an implantable power source must be developed.

Several possibilities are being pursued. They include thermoelectric devices that would convert body heat to electricity and piezoelectric devices that would convert motion (such as the movement of the rib cage during breathing) into electricity. A nuclear-powered battery may eventually be the answer, and considerable work is being done to develop one. The possibility of transmitting energy across the skin from an outside source is also under investigation.

But there is another pressing problem. When blood comes into contact with any surface other than the lining of blood vessels, its vital elements undergo gradual, progressive destruction. Efforts are being made to find suitable materials to line artificial hearts. This is no simple matter. The ideal material must not destroy blood elements; it must not cause clotting of blood; it must not cause allergic or toxic reactions, promote the development of cancer or interfere with the body's normal defense mechanism. It must also be tough and durable. For example, over a ten-year period, a diaphragm used in a pump of present design would be flexed almost 400 million times. Yet, under such stress, it could not break or leak.

Can these problems be solved? Many researchers are convinced they can be. A practical implantable artificial heart could save lives. It could eliminate the agony of finding a donor for a heart transplant. It might well be made in varied sizes to fit men, women and children.

Booster Hearts

Already one type of partial artificial heart, a booster heart, has begun to save lives. It does not take the place of the natural heart but takes over part of its job for hours, days or weeks to give the natural heart an opportunity to try to repair itself.

There are now several such devices. To understand their operation, recall that the left ventricle is the heart's main pumping chamber. It pumps oxygen-bearing blood to the rest of the body. Thus any kind of heart disease which affects the left ventricle can be critical. Failure of the left ventricle is most often the ultimate cause of death from heart disease.

Booster hearts are designed to help the failing left ventricle.

One such device, called a left ventricle pump, is a chamber about the size of a small apple, one side of which contains a flexible membrane. It is installed during open-heart surgery with connections to bypass blood around the left ventricle. When gas is pumped into the chamber, the membrane moves to the far side; as gas is withdrawn, the membrane goes back to its original side. With the membrane at rest, blood can flow in from the left atrium. When gas is pumped in, forcing the membrane to the other side, blood moves out into the body's arterial system. This type of booster heart does all the work of the left ventricle.

Another type assists, rather than replaces, the left ventricle. It is a rigid case containing a flexible inner lining. Through a flow of gas between case and lining, the lining is made to collapse and expand. The device is connected to the aorta so that all blood flowing through the body must pass through both the natural heart's left ventricle and the device. As the left ventricle pumps blood, the booster heart expands to receive it—and since the left ventricle is now pumping blood into an expanding chamber, it can do the pumping with relatively little work. Then the booster, activated by a pulse of gas, pumps the blood it has just received, sending it into the aorta and through the body.

Still another device is a balloon pump. It consists of a balloon at the end of a long tube which is attached to a pump. Balloon and tube are inserted into a leg artery and maneuvered upward into the aorta. The system is timed so that the balloon collapses just as the natural heart is expelling blood, thus providing an expanding space. Then the balloon is pumped up to help move blood through the body.

Assist devices are important steps on the way to a complete artificial heart, and they are also important in themselves.

As we have seen earlier, before the era of coronary care units and prompt detection and treatment for rhythm abnormalities, these abnormalities were the chief cause of death after heart attacks. Now the chief cause is cardiogenic shock—a grave lack of adequate circulation to body tissues because of reduction in heart output. If, during the critical period when the heart is so weakened that it cannot pump effectively, there could be assistance for it, a lightening of its load, the patient could be kept alive. Moreover, thanks to the partial rest, the heart might recover its pumping ability.

One of the very first patients on whom the balloon-assist device was used was a forty-five-year-old housewife who, after being hospitalized for a heart attack, went into cardiogenic shock. She was unconscious. Her blood pressure had almost disappeared. The outlook was for death within less than half an hour.

The balloon assist was inserted through a leg artery. As it began to function, greatly helping the heart to move blood through her body, she came out of shock. Five hours later, the pump could be stopped. The woman left the hospital alive and well. In a period of eighteen months in the same hospital, the balloon assist was used in twenty other patients. All were brought out of shock. About half recovered. The others died because the original damage from the heart attack was too great.

Perhaps these patients might have survived if an artificial heart had been available. But however desirable it may be, an artificial heart does not represent the ultimate solution to heart disease. The solution lies in further research to gain greater understanding of the causes of atherosclerosis and the ways of combating them. It also lies in immediate use by the public at large, with the guidance of the medical profession, of current knowledge about atherosclerosis in order to minimize the risk of coronary heart disease.

There have been many advances in treatment for all forms of heart disease—ways of saving many lives. Wisdom in their use is a responsibility of the medical profession—and the medical profession is aided in carrying out its responsibility by a public thoroughly acquainted with available measures and when they are best applied.

[19]

But Is It Really Heart Disease?

Real heart disease is a vast enough problem. But it has been estimated that as many as 20 million people in the United States, most of them men and many of them young, are bearing a needless burden. They think they have heart disease though they do not. Although they may have some of the symptoms—including chest pain, breathlessness, palpitation—there is nothing wrong with their hearts. But they live anxious, limited lives.

There are many different conditions with which coronary heart disease may be easily confused unless there is expert diagnosis.

One problem that can be mistaken for heart disease is irritability of the esophagus, called cardiospasm. The condition can produce chest pain similar to that of angina, a pain that frequently radiates upward, even to shoulders and upper arms. However, cardiospastic pain is usually briefer than real angina, comes on during rest and is often relieved by walking about.

A local problem in the chest itself, or in the shoulder girdle, may lead to pain on exertion, particularly when the chest muscles are used. An important distinguishing feature between such pain and true angina is that the latter is more likely to be triggered when leg muscles are used than when arm or chest muscles are.

It is possible to mistake gall-bladder disease for heart disease. A mild rib inflammation, or arthritis in the joints between rib and spine, also may mimic heart disease.

Bursitis, especially of the left shoulder, sometimes can act like coronary heart disease. So can neuralgia from spinal arthritis, particularly in the neck region. A study reported from one clinic showed that when 151 patients who thought they had heart disease were carefully checked, 35 had a cervical root syndrome. The syndrome—consisting of such symptoms as chest pain, numbness, tingling, weakness—stems from irritation of nerves in the neck area of the spine. Most commonly, poor posture is the cause. Sometimes, acute neck strain from a fall or other injury may be the cause. In many cases, posture correction is all that is needed to eliminate the symptoms. In others, a head-pulling (traction) device used at home may help.

Swallowing air, which becomes trapped in, and balloons, the intestinal tract, is a common cause of anginalike pain. The pain may spread to neck, shoulders and arms—and may be accompanied by trembling, sweating, weakness, breathlessness and pallor, much as in real heart disease. Often, a medication to help release entrapped air bubbles will provide relief.

Diaphragmatic hernia (also called hiatus hernia)—a condition in which part of the stomach protrudes up through the diaphragm into the chest—may cause anginalike pain. An X ray of the stomach can confirm the presence of diaphragmatic hernia. Sometimes, simple measures—such as elevation of the head of the bed and the use of antispasmodic medication—can alleviate the discomfort. When necessary, surgery can be used to overcome the problem.

Pain in the chest can come from pleurisy, an inflammation of the linings of the lungs. It can come from shingles, when nerves are irritated by a virus infection and produce acute pain. It has been known to come from food poisoning, from sleeping with arms or shoulders in unnatural position and from an unsuspected broken rib incurred during coughing.

Neurocirculatory asthenia is another condition often mistaken for heart disease. It can produce chest pain, dizziness, breathlessness, sweating, palpitation and profound fatigue. The cause is not definitely known, although most physicians believe there is a considerable emotional factor. The patient with neurocirculatory asthenia may be helped by psychotherapy or just by reassurance from physician and family. He may be helped, too, by graduated programs to increase the amount of exercise and activity he can tolerate, for he does not need to limit his activity.

Depression, or the blues, is a common emotional disturbance which can trigger anginalike pain. It sometimes does so under circumstances that would seem to make heart disease the obvious cause. For example, a forty-four-year-old man complained of chest pain which had begun several months before while he was engaged in heavy physical work. At first, he could get rid of the pain by resting for an hour. But then the pain began to persist both at work and at rest.

The results of a physical examination and an ECG were normal. Questioning revealed that the man not only had a despondent outlook on work and life but that he was waking earlier than usual, which is often an indication of depression. He was reassured that he had no heart disease and was given medication to combat the depression. Gradually, as his depression cleared, so did his chest pain.

Another patient, a forty-six-year-old woman, complained of pain "like a tight band across the chest." It had started several weeks before and was accentuated when she became emotionally upset. Physical findings and ECG were normal. When some gentle but penetrating questioning produced answers indicating a state of depression, she was treated for that. On her return for checkup, her chest pain had vanished.

Cardiac neurosis is common. It is easy enough for an emotionally troubled person who experiences a symptom such as chest pain, breathlessness or palpitation to become convinced he has heart disease. Many of the cardiac neurotics are not older people who might be expected to be somewhat concerned with their hearts but younger people between the ages of twenty and forty.

Many have become self-determined semi-invalids and in some cases even complete invalids.

An acute awareness of the action of the heart is common among cardiac neurotics. They often describe their heart action as pounding, loud enough to hear, rapid, irregular. They often become particularly aware of their heart actions at night while they are in bed, trying to fall asleep. The quieter the room, the more aware they are of their beating hearts. The experience can be alarming, and neurotics often find themselves fighting sleep, afraid they may not wake up again. They may suffer great fatigue in the morning and then may improve during the day if they become involved in activities that make them forget themselves. But as anxiety returns later in the day, fatigue and exhaustion recur.

Do you—or does anyone in the family—have what you suspect may be one symptom or several symptoms that could be caused by heart disease? By all means, get medical advice. As we have emphasized many times in this book, proper diagnosis is perhaps never more vital than when heart disease may be involved.

But don't assume that you do have heart disease—and don't assume that you don't. Consider again what we have noted in this chapter and also in Chapter 2 about the nature of symptoms. Then let your physician examine you thoroughly and determine, first of all, whether you have heart disease and, if you do, exactly what kind you have and what may best be done for it.

If you do not have heart disease, he can determine what it is you do have and what to do about that.

If, after your physician tells you that you do not have heart disease, you still continue to have lingering doubts, have his diagnosis confirmed by another physician.

Today, more effectively than ever before, the physician can treat heart disease when it exists. More effectively, too, than ever before, he can determine when it does and does not exist.

We hope this book has helped you to understand more completely how your physician goes about diagnosis and why he can reassure you when he finds that there is no evidence of heart disease. For understanding this can be as important as understanding the strides of modern medicine and surgery in diagnosing and treating heart disease when it does exist. There is no reason why a fancied disease should impose needless restrictions and anxieties on you or any member of your family—just as there is no reason that, if you have heart disease, you should assume your life is over. Though real heart disease is a serious problem, there is much that can now be done to minimize its risks and to combat it.

Appendix

The American Heart Association's

FAT-CONTROLLED, LOW-CHOLESTEROL MEAL PLAN*

This plan is mainly for adults who have a family history of heart disease, or who may have increased their risks through a regular diet high in saturated fat and cholesterol. Children and adolescents, especially from susceptible families, can also benefit from this meal plan by forming early in life tastes for food that may protect them from heart disease when they reach adulthood.

The *types* of food recommended here are suitable for most people from childhood through maturity. The *amounts* of food specified in the food list, however, are recommended mainly for the average adult. Nutritional needs differ during growth periods of infants, children and adolescents, and during pregnancy and breast feeding; at these times, the amounts of food to be eaten should be regulated by a physician.

To use this plan, simply select, every day, foods from each of the basic food groups in lists 1 to 5, and follow the recommendations for the number and size of servings.

* This plan, with only slight modifications of position and wording, has been reprinted from *The Way to a Man's Heart,* a leaflet published by the American Heart Association (© American Heart Association, 1968).

241

1. MEAT, POULTRY, FISH, DRIED BEANS AND PEAS, NUTS, EGGS

One serving: 3–4 ounces of cooked meat or fish (not including bone or fat) or 3–4 ounces of a vegetable listed here. Use 2 or more servings (a total of 6–8 ounces) daily.

RECOMMENDED

Chicken • turkey • veal • fish • in most of your meat meals for the week.

Beef • lamb • pork • ham • in no more than 5 meals per week. Choose lean ground meat and lean cuts of meat • trim all visible fat before cooking • bake, broil, roast or stew so that you can discard the fat which cooks out of the meat.

Nuts and dried beans and peas: Kidney beans • lima beans • baked beans • lentils • chick peas (garbanzos) • split peas • are high in vegetable protein and may be used in place of meat occasionally.

Egg whites as desired.

AVOID OR USE SPARINGLY

Duck • goose

Shellfish: clams • crab • lobster • oysters • scallops • shrimp • are low in fat but high in cholesterol. Use a 4-ounce serving as a substitute for meat no more than twice a week.

Heavily marbled and fatty meats • spare ribs • mutton • frankfurters • sausages • fatty hamburgers • bacon • luncheon meats.

Organ meats: liver • kidney • heart • sweetbreads • are very high in cholesterol. Since liver is very rich in vitamins and iron, it should not be eliminated from the diet completely. Use a 4-ounce serving in a meat meal no more than once a week.

Egg yolks: limit to 3 per week, including eggs used in cooking.

Cakes, batters, sauces and other foods containing egg yolks.

2. VEGETABLES AND FRUIT (Fresh, Frozen or Canned)

One serving: ½ cup. Use at least 4 servings daily.

RECOMMENDED

One serving should be a source of Vitamin C:
Broccoli • cabbage (raw) • tomatoes.

Berries • cantaloupe • grapefruit (or juice) • mango • melon • orange (or juice) • papaya • strawberries • tangerines.

One serving should be a source of Vitamin A—dark green leafy or yellow vegetables, or yellow fruits:
Broccoli • carrots • chard • chicory • escarole • greens (beet, collard, dandelion, mustard, turnip) • kale • peas • rutabagas • spinach • string beans • sweet potatoes and yams • watercress • winter squash • yellow corn.

Apricots • cantaloupe • mango • papaya.

Other vegetables and fruits are also very nutritious; they should be eaten in salads, main dishes, snacks and desserts, *in addition* to the recommended daily allowances of high vitamin A and C vegetables and fruits. If you must limit your calories, use a serving of potatoes, yellow corn or fresh or frozen cooked lima beans in place of a bread serving.

AVOID OR USE SPARINGLY

Olives and avocados are very high in fat calories and should be used in moderation.

3. BREADS AND CEREALS (Whole grain, enriched or restored)

One serving of bread: 1 slice. One serving of cereal: ½ cup, cooked; 1 cup, cold, with skimmed milk. Use at least 4 servings daily.

RECOMMENDED

Breads made with a minimum of saturated fat:
White enriched (including raisin bread) • whole wheat • English muffins • French bread • Italian bread • oatmeal bread • pumpernickel • rye bread.

Biscuits, muffins, and griddle cakes made at home, using an allowed liquid oil as shortening.

Cereal (hot and cold) • rice • melba toast • matzo • pretzels.

Pasta: macaroni • noodles (except egg noodles) • spaghetti.

AVOID OR USE SPARINGLY

Butter rolls • commercial biscuits, muffins, doughnuts, sweet rolls, cakes, crackers • egg bread, cheese bread • commercial mixes containing dried eggs and whole milk.

4. MILK PRODUCTS

One serving: 8 ounces (1 cup). Buy only skimmed milk that has been fortified with Vitamins A and D. Daily servings: children up to twelve, 3 or more cups; teen-agers, 4 or more cups; adults, 2 or more cups.

RECOMMENDED

Milk products that are low in dairy fats:

Fortified skimmed (nonfat) milk and fortified skimmed milk powder • low-fat milk. The label on the container should show that the milk is fortified with Vitamins A and D. The word "fortified" alone is not enough.

Buttermilk made from skimmed milk • yogurt made from skimmed milk • canned evaporated skimmed milk • cocoa made with low-fat milk.

Cheeses made from skimmed or partially skimmed milk, such as cottage cheese, creamed or uncreamed (uncreamed, preferably) • farmer's, baker's or hoop cheese • mozzarella and sapsago cheeses.

AVOID OR USE SPARINGLY

Whole milk and whole milk products:

Chocolate milk • canned whole milk • ice cream • all creams, including sour, half and half, whipped • whole-milk yogurt.

Nondairy cream substitutes usually contain coconut oil, which is very high in saturated fat.

Cheeses made from cream or whole milk.

Butter.

5. FATS AND OILS (Polyunsaturated)

An individual allowance should include about 2–4 tablespoons daily (depending on how many calories you can afford) in the form of margarine, salad dressing and shortening.

RECOMMENDED

Margarines, liquid oil shortenings, salad dressings and mayonnaise containing any of these polyunsaturated vegetable oils:
Corn oil • cottonseed oil • safflower oil • sesame seed oil • soybean oil • sunflower seed oil.

Margarines and other products high in polyunsaturates can usually be identified by their label, which lists a recommended *liquid* vegetable oil as the *first* ingredient, and one or more partially hydrogenated vegetable oils as additional ingredients.

Diet margarines are low in calories because they are low in fat. Therefore it takes twice as much diet margarine to supply the polyunsaturates contained in a recommended margarine.

AVOID OR USE SPARINGLY

Solid fats and shortenings:
Butter • lard • salt pork fat • meat fat • completely hydrogenated margarines and vegetable shortenings • products containing coconut oil.

Peanut oil and olive oil may be used occasionally for flavor, but they are low in polyunsaturates and do not take the place of the recommended oils.

6. DESSERTS, BEVERAGES, SNACKS, CONDIMENTS

The foods on this list are acceptable because they are low in saturated fat and cholesterol. If you have eaten your daily allowance from the first five lists, however, these foods will be in excess of your nutritional needs, and many of them also may exceed your calorie limits for maintaining a desirable weight. If you must limit your calories, limit your portions of the foods on this list as well.

Moderation should be observed especially in the use of alcoholic drinks, ice milk, sherbet, sweets and bottled drinks.

ACCEPTABLE

Low in calories or no calories:
Fresh fruit and fruit canned without sugar • tea, coffee (no cream), cocoa powder • water ices • gelatin • fruit whip • puddings made with nonfat milk • sweets and bottled drinks made with artificial sweeteners • vinegar, mustard, ketchup, herbs, spices.

High in calories:
Frozen or canned fruit with sugar added • jelly, jam, marmalade, honey • pure sugar candy such as gum drops, hard candy, mint patties (not chocolate) • imitation ice cream made with safflower oil • cakes, pies, cookies and puddings made with polyunsaturated fat in place of solid shortening • angel food cake • nuts, especially walnuts • nonhydrogenated peanut butter • bottled drinks • fruit drinks • ice milk • sherbet • wine, beer, whiskey.

AVOID OR USE SPARINGLY

Coconut and coconut oil • commercial cakes, pies, cookies and mixes • frozen cream pies • commercially fried foods such as potato chips and other deep-fried snacks • whole-milk puddings • chocolate pudding (high in cocoa butter and therefore high in saturated fat) • ice cream.

A Dictionary of Heart Terms

Adrenalin (ad-ren'al-in). A secretion of the adrenal glands, two small glands above the kidneys. The secretion, which is also called epinephrine, constricts the small blood vessels (arterioles), increases the rate of the heart beat and raises blood pressure.

Aneurysm (an'you-rizm). A saclike bulging of the heart or of the wall of a vein or artery, which may result from weakening by disease or an abnormality present at birth.

Angina pectoris (an'jin-a or an-jy'na pek'to-ris). Chest pain caused by an inadequate blood supply to the heart muscle. It commonly results from narrowing of the arteries (coronaries) that supply the heart muscle.

Angiocardiography (an'jee-oh-kar-dee-og'ra-fee). An X-ray examination of the heart and great blood vessels after an opaque fluid, or dye, is injected into the blood stream.

Anoxia (an-ok'see-a). Lack of oxygen. This most often occurs when blood supply to a part of the body is cut off completely, and it results in death of the affected tissue. For example, a part of the heart muscle may die when its blood (and therefore oxygen) supply has been stopped by a clot in the artery supplying that area.

Anticoagulant (an'tee-koh-ag'you-lant). A drug capable of slowing the clotting of blood. When used where a clot has obstructed a blood vessel, it does not dissolve the clot but helps prevent new clot formation and enlargement of existing clots.

Antihypertensive agent (an'tee-hy-per-ten'siv). A drug used to lower blood pressure.

Anxiety (ang-zy'i-tee). A feeling of

248

apprehension the source of which is not recognized.

Aorta (ay-or'ta). The main trunk artery of the body. It begins at the base of the heart, where it receives blood from the lower left heart chamber (left ventricle); arches up over the heart much like a cane handle; then passes down through the chest and abdomen in front of the spine. From the aorta many arteries branch off transporting blood to all parts of the body except the lungs.

Aortic arch (ay-or'tik). The part of the aorta which curves up over the heart like a cane handle.

Aortic insufficiency. Improper closing of the valve between the aorta and the heart's lower left chamber or ventricle, permitting some backflow of blood from the aorta into the ventricle.

Aortic stenosis (ste-noh'sis). A narrowing of the valve opening between the lower left heart chamber and the aorta. The narrowing may result from scar-tissue formation after rheumatic fever or other causes.

Aortic valve. The valve at the junction of the aorta and lower left heart chamber. Formed by three cup-shaped membranes, it permits blood to flow from the heart into the aorta and prevents backflow.

Aortography (ay-or-tog'ra-fee). X-ray examination of the aorta and its main branches after injection of a dye to make the structures visible.

Apex (ay'peks). The blunt rounded end of the heart, directed downward and to the left.

Arrhythmia (ah-rith'mee-a). An abnormal rhythm of the heartbeat.

Arterial blood (ar-tee'ree-al). Oxy-genated blood. The blood receives its oxygen in the lungs and then passes from the lungs to the left side or. the heart through the pulmonary veins. From there it is pumped into the arteries, which carry it to all parts of the body.

Arterioles (ar-tee'ree-ohlz). The smallest arterial vessels (about 1/125 inch or 0.2 mm. in diameter). They conduct blood from the arteries to the capillaries, vessels through which oxygen and nutritive materials can pass into the tissues.

Arteriosclerosis (ar-tee'ree-oh-skle-roh'sis). Hardening of the arteries. Arteriosclerosis is a broad term which includes varied conditions that cause artery walls to become thick and hard and lose their elasticity. See *Atherosclerosis*.

Artery (ar'ter-ee). A blood vessel which transports blood away from the heart to some part of the body.

Atheroma (ath-er-oh'ma). A deposit of fatty and other substances in the inner lining of an artery wall. The plural for atheroma is atheromata (ath-er-oh-mah'ta).

Atherosclerosis (ath'er-oh-skle-roh'-sis). A type of arteriosclerosis in which the inner layer of the artery wall is made thick and irregular by deposits of fatty substance. These deposits (atheromata) project and thus decrease the internal diameter of the artery.

Atrial septum (ay'tree-al). The wall that divides the left and right upper chambers of the heart, which are called atria.

Atrio-ventricular bundle (ay'tree-oh-ven-trik'you-lar). A bundle of specialized muscle fibers, also called the A-V bundle and the *Bundle of His*. It runs from a small mass of muscular fibers (atrio-ventricular node) between the upper heart chambers down to the lower chambers. It conducts impulses from the atrio-ventricular node for the rhythmic beat of the heart.

Atrio-ventricular node. A small mass of special muscular fibers at the base of the wall between the two upper heart chambers. Electrical impulses which control the heart rhythm are generated by the pacemaker, a small mass of special cells in the right upper chamber of the heart. The impulses are conducted through the muscle fibers of the right upper chamber to the atrio-ventricular node, and then to the lower chambers, by the *Atrio-ventricular bundle* or *Bundle of His*.

Atrio-ventricular valves. The valves, one in each side of the heart, between upper and lower chambers. The one in the right side is called the tricuspid valve, and the one in the left side is called the mitral valve.

Atrium (ay'tree-um). One of the two upper chambers of the heart. The right atrium receives "used" or unoxygenated blood from the body; the left atrium receives oxygenated blood from the lungs.

Auricle (aw're-kul). Another name for the upper chamber in each side of the heart. See *Atrium*.

Auscultation (aws-kul-tay'shun). The act of listening, usually with a stethoscope, to sounds within the body.

Autonomic nervous system (aw-to-nom'ik). The system which controls the functioning of or-gans and tissues not under voluntary control, such as the glands, heart and smooth muscles. It is sometimes called the involuntary nervous system or vegetative nervous system.

Bacterial endocarditis (bak-tee'ree-al en'doh-kar-dy'tis). An inflammation of the inner layer of the heart, most often the lining of the heart valves, caused by bacteria. It is most frequently a complication of an infectious disease, operation or injury.

Ballistocardiogram (bal-lis'toh-kar'-dee-oh-gram). A recording of movements of the body produced by the beating of the heart. The instrument used for the recording is called a ballistocardiograph.

Bicuspid valve (by-kus'pid). More often called the mitral valve. It is a valve of two cusps, or triangular segments, located between the upper and lower chamber in the left side of the heart.

Blood pressure. The pressure of the blood in the arteries. Blood pressure when the heart muscle is contracted (systole) is called systolic. Blood pressure when the heart muscle is relaxed between beats (diastole) is called diastolic.

Blue babies. Babies whose skin has a bluish look (cyanosis) because of insufficient oxygen in the arterial blood. This is often the result of a heart defect but may have other causes, such as impaired respiration or premature birth.

Bradycardia (brad-ee-kar'dee-a). An abnormally slow heart rate—generally, anything below 60 beats per minute.

Bundle of His (hiss: named after Wilhelm His, German anatomist). A bundle of specialized muscular fibers running from the atrio-ventricular node between the upper chambers of the heart down to the lower chambers. It conducts impulses for the rhythmic heartbeat from the atrio-ventricular node. Also called *atrio-ventricular bundle,* or A-V bundle.

Capillary (kap'i-lar-ee). A narrow vessel with a wall made up of a single layer of cells through which oxygen and nutritive materials move to the tissues and carbon dioxide and waste products are admitted from the tissues into the blood stream.

Cardiac (kar'dee-ak). (Adj.) Pertaining to the heart. Sometimes used (n.) to refer to anyone who has heart disease.

Cardiac cycle. One total heartbeat, or complete contraction and relaxation of the heart.

Cardiac output. The amount of blood pumped by the heart per minute.

Cardiovascular (kar'dee-o-vas'kyou-lar). Pertaining to the heart and blood vessels.

Cardiovascular-renal disease (ree'-nal). Disease involving the heart, blood vessels and kidneys.

Carditis (kar-dy'tis). Inflammation of the heart.

Carotid arteries (kah-rot'id). The left and right common carotid arteries are the main vessels supplying the head and neck. Each has two main branches, external carotid and internal carotid.

Carotid body. A small mass of cells and nerve endings in the carotid sinus or branching point in the arteries supplying the head and neck. The carotid body is sensitive to chemical changes in the blood and in response to these changes causes changes in breathing rate and other functions. For example, when oxygen content of the blood is reduced, the carotid body triggers an increase in breathing rate.

Carotid sinus (sy'nus). A slight dilation at the point where the internal carotid artery branches from the common carotid artery. The carotid sinus contains nerve-end organs which are sensitive to changes in blood pressure and in response to these changes cause a change in heartbeat rate.

Catheter (kath'e-ter). A cardiac catheter is a thin tube of plastic or other material which is inserted in a vein or artery, usually in the arm, and pushed into the heart. It is used to take blood samples or pressure readings inside the heart chambers.

Catheterization (kath'e-ter-i-zay'-shun). In cardiology, the process of examining the heart by introducing a catheter, or thin tube, into a vein or artery and moving it into the heart.

Cerebral vascular accident (ser'e-bral vas'kyou-lar). Also called cerebrovascular accident, or *stroke.* It denotes impeded blood supply to the brain. It may be caused by (1) formation of a blood clot in a vessel supplying the brain (cerebral thrombosis); (2) rupture of a blood-vessel wall (cerebral hemorrhage); (3) blockage of a brain blood vessel by a clot or other material formed elsewhere which moves to the cerebral vessel (cerebral embolism); (4) pressure on a blood vessel—by a tumor, for example.

Cerebrovascular (ser'e-broh-vas'kyou-lar). Pertaining to blood vessels in the brain.

Chemotherapy (kem-oh-ther'a-pee). The treatment of disease by chemicals.

Cholesterol (koh-les'ter-ol). A fatlike substance found in animal tissue. In blood tests, the normal level of Americans is thought to be between 180 and 230 milligrams per 100 cubic centimeters. A higher level is often associated with risk of coronary atherosclerosis.

Chorea (koh-ree'a). Also called St. Vitus's dance, or Sydenham's chorea. Irregular, involuntary twitching of muscles. Sometimes associated with rheumatic fever.

Circulatory (ser'kyou-la-to-ree). Pertaining to the heart, blood vessels and circulation of blood.

Claudication (klaw-di-kay'shun). Pain and limping or lameness caused by impaired circulation in the blood vessels of the limbs.

Clubbed fingers (klubd). Fingers with short, broad tips and overhanging nails. The condition is sometimes seen in children with certain congenital heart defects.

Coagulation (koh-ag-you-lay'shun). The changing of a liquid to a thickened or solid material; formation of a clot.

Coarctation of the aorta (koh-ark-tay'shun). A narrowing of the aorta, or main trunk artery of the body. One type of congenital heart defect.

Collateral circulation (ko-lat'er-al). Blood circulation through nearby smaller vessels when a main vessel becomes blocked.

Commissurotomy (kom-i-shur-ot'o-mee). An operation to enlarge the opening in a heart valve which has been narrowed by scar tissue. The operation is often used in patients with rheumatic heart disease.

Compensation. An adjustment made by the circulatory system to counteract some abnormality. It may be an adjustment in size of heart or rate of beat to counterbalance a defect in structure or function.

Congenital anomaly (kon-jen'i-tal a-nom'a-lee). An abnormality present at birth.

Congestive heart failure. A condition that occurs when the heart cannot pump out effectively all the blood that returns to it, and blood backs up in veins leading to the heart. Congestion, or fluid accumulation, may occur in various parts of the body, such as lungs, legs, abdomen, as a result of the heart's failure to maintain normal circulation.

Constriction. Narrowing of some type. For example, vaso-constriction indicates a narrowing of the internal diameter of blood vessels caused by contraction of muscles in the vessel walls.

Constrictive pericarditis (per'i-kar-dy'tis). Shrinking and thickening of the heart's outer sac which interferes with normal expansion and contraction of the heart.

Coronary arteries (kor'oh-nay-ree). The two arteries which arise from the aorta and arch down over the top of the heart, conducting blood to the heart muscle.

Coronary atherosclerosis (ath'er-oh-skle-roh'sis). Also called coronary heart disease, this is an irregular thickening of the inner lining of the walls of the coronary arteries so that the channel through which blood flows to feed the heart muscle is narrowed and the flow reduced.

Coronary occlusion (ok-kloo'zhun). An obstruction, such as a clot in a branch of a coronary artery, hindering the flow of blood to some part of the heart muscle. For lack of blood supply, this part of the muscle dies. Sometimes called coronary heart attack, or heart attack.

Coronary thrombosis (throm-boh'-sis). Formation of a clot in a coronary artery branch. A form of coronary occlusion.

Cor pulmonale (kor' pul-moh-nal'ee). Heart disease caused by disease of the lungs, or of blood vessels in the lungs, increasing resistance to blood flow through the lungs.

Cyanosis (sy-a-noh'sis). Blueness of the skin caused by insufficient oxygen in the blood.

Cytologic (sy-toh-loj'ik). Pertaining to cells and their anatomy, physiology, chemistry and pathology.

Decompensation. Inability of the heart to maintain adequate circulation, usually leading to fluid accumulation in tissues. A person is said to be decompensated when the heart fails to maintain normal circulation.

Defibrillator (dee-fi'bri-lay-tor). Any measure, such as an electric shock, which stops uncoordinated contraction of the heart muscle and restores normal heartbeat.

Diastole (dy-as'toh-lee). The period of relaxation of the heart in each heartbeat.

Digitalis (dij-i-tal'is). A drug made from leaves of the foxglove that strengthens heart-muscle contraction, slows the contraction rate and improves efficiency of the heart so that fluid may be eliminated from body tissues.

Dilation. Enlargement or stretching of heart or blood vessels.

Diuresis (dy-you-ree'sis). Increased excretion of urine.

Diuretic (dy-you-ret'ik). A medication which promotes excretion of urine.

Ductus arteriosus (duk'tus ar-tee'ree-oh'sis). In the fetus, a small duct between the artery leaving the left side of the heart (aorta) and the artery leaving the right side of the heart (pulmonary artery). Normally, the duct closes soon after birth. If it does not close, the condition is known as *patent*, or open, *ductus arteriosus*.

Dyspnea (disp-nee'a). Difficult or labored breathing.

ECG. See *Electocardiogram*.

Edema (e-dee'ma). Swelling due to abnormal collection of fluids in body tissues.

Effort Syndrome (sin'drohm). A group of symptoms (easy fatigue, rapid heartbeat, sighing breaths, dizziness) that do not stem from disease and are out of proportion to the amount of effort expended.

EKG. See *Electrocardiogram*.

Electric cardiac pacemaker. An electric device that discharges rhythmic electrical impulses to control beating of the heart.

Electrocardiogram (e-lek-troh-kar'dee-oh-gram). Also called EKG and ECG. A record of the electric currents produced by the heart.

Electrocardiograph (e-lek-troh-kar'

dee-oh-graf). An instrument that records the electric currents produced by the heart.

Embolism (em'boh-lizm). The blocking of a blood vessel by a clot or other material carried in the blood.

Embolus (em'boh-lus). A clot or other material such as air or fat carried in the blood stream to a small vessel, where it lodges and blocks flow.

Endocarditis (en'doh-kar-dy'tis). Inflammation of the inner layer of the heart (the endocardium), usually associated with acute rheumatic fever or some other infection.

Endocardium (en-doh-kar'dee-um). A thin smooth membrane forming the inner surface of the heart.

Endothelium (en-doh-thee'lee-um). The thin lining of blood vessels.

Enzyme (en'zym). A complex chemical which speeds up specific biochemical processes in the body. Many enzymes are present in living organisms.

Epicardium (ep-i-kar'dee-um). The outer layer of the heart wall.

Epinephrine (ep-i-nef'rin). A secretion of the adrenal glands, which are located above the kidneys. Also called adrenalin, the secretion constricts small blood vessels, increases heartbeat rate, and raises blood pressure.

Erythrocyte (e-rith'roh-syt). A red blood cell.

Essential hypertension (hy-per-ten' shun). Elevated or high blood pressure not caused by kidney or other evident disease.

Etiology (ee-tee-ol'oh-jee). What is known about the causes of a disease.

Extracorporeal circulation (eks-tra-kor-po'ree-al). Circulation of blood outside the body, as by a heart-lung machine during surgery inside the heart.

Extrasystole (eks-tra-sis'toh-lee). A heart contraction which occurs prematurely and interrupts normal rhythm.

Eyeground (i'ground). The inside of the back part of the eye, also called the fundus, which can be seen through the pupil. Eyeground examination helps assess changes in blood vessels.

Femoral artery (fem'or-al). Main vessel supplying blood to the leg.

Fibrillation (fy-bri-lay'shun). Uncoordinated contractions, virtually mere twitchings, of the heart muscle.

Fibrin (fy'brin). A protein material which forms the essential part of a blood clot.

Fibrinogen (fy-brin'oh-jen). A soluble protein in the blood which can be converted by certain enzymes into the insoluble protein of a clot.

Fibrinolysin (fy-bri-nohl'is-in). An enzyme which makes coagulated blood liquid again.

Fibrinolytic (fy-brin-oh-lit'ik). Having ability to dissolve a blood clot.

Fluoroscope (floo-oh'roh-skohp). An instrument which passes X rays through the body onto a flourescent screen, where the shadows of internal organs can be seen.

Fluoroscopy (floo-or-os'koh-pee). The examination of internal structures by means of the fluoroscope.

Fundus. The inside of the back part of the eye, also called the eyeground, which can be seen through the pupil. Examination of the fundus is useful in assessing changes in blood vessels.

Gallop rhythm. An extra heart sound which, when the heart rate is fast, resembles a horse's gallop. It may or may not be significant.

Ganglion (gang'glee-on). A mass of nerve cells which acts as a nerve system center.

Ganglionic blocking agents (gang-glee-on'ik). Drugs that stop the transmission of nerve impulses at the nerve centers (ganglia). Some of these agents are used in treating high blood pressure.

Genetics (je-net'iks). The study of heredity.

Heart block. Partial or complete interference with the conduction of electrical impulses of the heart. Rhythms of upper and lower heart chambers may then become dissociated.

Heart-lung machine. A machine which pumps and oxygenates blood so that blood can be diverted from the heart while it is opened for surgery.

Hemodynamics (hee'moh-dy-nam'-iks). The study of blood flow and the forces involved.

Hemoglobin (hee'moh-gloh'bin). The pigment of the red blood cells which carries oxygen. When it absorbs oxygen in the lungs, it is bright red. After it has given up oxygen to body tissues, it is purple.

Hemorrhage (hem'or-ij). Loss of blood from a vessel. In an external hemorrhage, blood escapes from the body; in an internal hemorrhage, the blood moves into tissues surrounding the ruptured vessel.

Heparin (hep'a-rin). An anticoagulant drug which helps to keep blood from clotting.

Hypercholesteremia (hy-per-koh-les-ter-ee'mee-a). An excess of the fatty substance, cholesterol, in the blood.

Hyperlipemia (hy-per-ly-pee'mee-a). An excess of fats, or lipids, in the blood.

Hypertension (hy-per-ten'shun). Also called high blood pressure. An elevation of blood pressure above normal range.

Hyperthyroidism (hy-per-thy'roid-izm). Excessive activity of the thyroid gland, which may result in speed-up of the heartbeat rate.

Hypertrophy (hy-per'troh-fee). Enlargement of an organ or tissue resulting from an increase in size of the cells that compose it.

Hypotension (hy-poh-ten'shun). Also called low blood pressure. A level of blood pressure below normal range.

Hypothermia (hy-poh-ther'mee-a). Cooling of body temperature (usually to 86 to 88 degrees F.) to slow down metabolic processes during heart surgery. In this cooled state, body tissues need less oxygen.

Hypothyroidism (hy-poh-thy'roid-izm). Excessive activity of the thyroid gland, resulting in slowing down of many body processes, including heart rate.

Hypoxia (hy-pok'see-a). A less than normal amount of oxygen in organs and tissues of the body.

Iatrogenic heart disease (i'at-roh-jen-ik). Literally means "caused by the doctor." It usually refers to a patient's belief he has heart disease, inferred from a physician's actions, manner or discussion.

Iliac artery (il'ee-ak). A large artery

carrying blood to the pelvis and legs.

Incompetent valve. Any heart valve which does not close properly, thus allowing blood to leak back in the wrong direction.

Infarct (in-farkt'). An area of tissue damaged or dead as a result of inadequate blood supply. A myocardial infarct indicates an area of heart muscle damaged or killed by insufficient blood flow through a coronary artery which normally supplies it.

Innominate artery (in-nom'i-nate). One of the largest branches of the aorta. It arises from the arch of the aorta and divides to form the common carotid artery and the right subclavian artery.

Insufficiency. An incompetency. Thus, a valvular insufficiency indicates the improper closing of a valve allowing backflow of blood in the wrong direction. A myocardial insufficiency indicates inability of the heart muscle to pump normally.

Interatrial septum (in-ter-ay'tree-al). The wall dividing left and right upper chambers of the heart.

Interventricular septum (in-ter-ven-trik'you-lar). The wall dividing left and right lower chambers of the heart.

Intima (in'ti-ma). The innermost layer of a blood vessel.

Ischemia (is-kee'mee-a). A usually temporary deficiency of blood in some part of the body, often caused by a constriction or obstruction in a blood vessel.

Jugular veins (jug'you-lar). The veins which return blood from head and neck to the heart.

Linoleic acid (lin-oh-lay'ik). A component of many unsaturated fats. It occurs in oils from many plants. A diet high in linoleic acid tends to reduce the level of cholesterol in the blood.

Lipid (lip'id). Fat.

Lipoprotein (lip-oh-proh'tee-in). A complex of fat and protein molecules.

Lumen (lyou'men). The passageway or channel inside a tubular organ.

Malignant hypertension (mah-lig'-nant hy-per-ten'shun). A severe form of high blood pressure which, unless controlled, runs a rapid course and damages blood-vessel walls in the kidneys, eyes and elsewhere.

Mercurial diuretic (mer-kyou'ree-al di-you-ret'ik). A compound containing mercury that is used to promote elimination of excess fluids from the body through increased exertion of urine.

Metabolism (me-tab'oh-lizm). A term that refers to all chemical changes which occur to substances within the body.

Mitral insufficiency (my'tral). Improper closing of the mitral valve between upper and lower chambers of left side of heart, permitting blood to flow back in the wrong direction. Sometimes the result of scar tissue formed after a rheumatic-fever infection.

Mitral stenosis (ste-noh'sis). Narrowing of the valve opening between upper and lower chambers in the left side of the heart. Sometimes the result of scar tissue formed after rheumatic-fever infection.

Mitral valve. Also called *bicuspid valve.* A valve with two cusps or triangular segments, located between upper and lower chambers in the left side of the heart.

Mitral valvulotomy (my'tral val-vyou-lot'o-mee). An operation to enlarge the opening in the valve between upper and lower chambers in the left side of the heart when the opening is so reduced as to impair blood flow.

Mono-unsaturated fat (mon-oh-un-sat'you-rayt-ed). A fat so made up chemically that it can absorb additional hydrogen but not so much hydrogen as a polyunsaturated fat. Such fat in the diet has little effect on the level of cholesterol in the blood. One example of a mono-unsaturated fat is olive oil.

Murmur. An unusual or abnormal heart sound. It is sometimes significant and of diagnostic value. Many murmurs, however, have no importance.

Myocardial infarction (my-oh-kar'-dee-al). Damage or death of an area of heart muscle from reduced blood supply to the area.

Myocardial insufficiency. Inability of the heart muscle to maintain normal circulation.

Myocarditis (my'oh-kar-dy'tis). Inflammation of the heart muscle.

Myocardium (my-oh-kar'dee-um). The muscular wall of the heart.

Neurocirculatory asthenia (nyou-roh-ser'ku-la-to-ree as-thee'nee-a). A complex of symptoms, often including fatigue, dizziness, shortness of breath, rapid heartbeat and nervousness. Also called *effort syndrome* and *soldier's heart.*

Neurogenic (nyou-roh-jen'ik). Originating in the nervous system.

Normotensive. Characterized by normal blood pressure.

Open-heart surgery. Surgery carried out on the opened heart while blood is diverted through a heart-lung machine.

Organic heart disease. Heart disease resulting from some structural abnormality in the heart or circulatory system.

Pacemaker. (1) A small mass of special cells in the right upper chamber of the heart which produce the electrical impulses that initiate heart contractions. Also called *sino-atrial node* or *S-A node.* (2) An electrical device that can substitute for the defective natural pacemaker and control beating of the heart by a series of rhythmic electrical discharges.

Palpitation. A fluttering of the heart or an abnormal rhythm or rate experienced by the person himself.

Parasympathetic nervous system. A part of the autonomic, or involuntary, nervous system. Stimulation of various parasympathetic nerves causes pupils of the eyes to contract and the heart to beat more slowly, as well as producing other nonvoluntary reactions.

Paroxysmal tachycardia (par-ok-siz'-mal tak-ee-kar'dee-a). An episode of rapid heart beating which begins and ends suddenly.

Patent ductus arteriosus (pay'tent duk'tus ar-tee'ree-oh'sis). A heart defect in which a small duct between the aorta and the pulmonary artery which normally closes soon after birth remains open. ("Patent" means open.) As a result of the duct's failure to close, blood from both sides, instead of just one side, of the heart is pumped into the pulmonary artery and into the lungs.

Pathogenesis (path-oh-jen'e-sis). The events leading to development of disease.

Pathology. The study of the nature of disease and the changes in structure and function it produces.

Percussion. Finger-tapping of the body as a help in diagnosing the condition of parts beneath by the sound obtained.

Pericarditis (per'i-kar-dy'tis). Inflammation of the sac which surrounds the heart.

Pericardium (per-i-kar'dee-um). The thin sac which surrounds the heart.

Peripheral resistance (pe-rif'er-al). The resistance offered by the arterioles and capillaries to blood flow from arteries to veins. An increase in peripheral resistance causes an increase in blood pressure.

Pharmacology. The science which deals with drugs in all their aspects.

Phlebitis (fleh-by'tis). Inflammation of a vein, often in the leg.

Plasma (plaz'ma). The liquid, cell-free portion of uncoagulated blood. It differs from serum, which is the fluid part of blood obtained after coagulation.

Polycythemia (pol-ee-sy-thee'mee-a). An abnormal blood condition in which there is an excessive number of red cells.

Polyunsaturated fat (pol-ee-un-sat'-you-rayt-ed). A fat chemically composed so it can absorb additional hydrogen. Such a fat is usually a liquid oil of vegetable origin, such as corn or safflower oil. A diet with high polyunsaturated fat content tends to reduce the level of cholesterol in the blood.

Pressor (pres'or). A substance which raises blood pressure and speeds the heartbeat.

Prophylaxis (proh-fi-lak'sis). Preventive treatment.

Psychosomatic (sy-koh-soh-mat'ik). Pertaining to the influence of the mind and emotions on body functioning.

Pulmonary artery (pul'moh-nay-ree). The large artery that carries unoxygenated blood from the lower right chamber of the heart to the lungs.

Pulmonary circulation. The circulation of the blood through the lungs—from right lower heart chamber to lungs and back to left upper heart chamber.

Pulmonary valve. The valve, formed by three cup-shaped membranes, at the junction of pulmonary artery and right lower heart chamber.

Pulmonary veins. Four veins (two from each lung) which carry oxygenated blood from lungs to left upper chamber of the heart.

Pulse. The expansion and contraction of an artery which may be felt with a finger. The contractions of the artery walls correspond to the contractions of the heart and so are indications of heartbeat.

Pulsus alternans (pul'sus awl-ter'nans). A pulse in which weak and strong beats regularly alternate.

Regurgitation. The backward flow of blood through a defective valve.

Renal (ree'nal). Pertaining to the kidney.

Renal circulation. The circulation of blood through the kidneys.

Renal hypertension. High blood pressure caused by damage or disease of the kidneys.

Rheumatic fever (roo-mat'ik). A disease, most frequent in childhood, which may develop a few weeks after a streptococcal infection. It may be marked by one or more of such symptoms as fever, sore, swollen joints, skin rash, or involuntary twitching of muscles (*chorea* or St. Vitus's dance).

Rheumatic heart disease. The damage done to the heart, particularly the heart valves, by one or more attacks of rheumatic fever. The valves may be scarred so they no longer open and close properly.

S-A node. A small mass of specialized cells in the heart's upper right chamber which originate the electrical pulses that produce contractions of the heart. Also known as *sino-atrial node* or *pacemaker.*

Saturated fat. A fat so constituted chemically that it cannot absorb any more hydrogen. Usually the solid fats of animal origin such as those in milk, butter, meat, etc., are saturated. A diet high in saturated fat tends to increase levels of cholesterol in the blood.

Sclerosis (skle-roh'sis). Hardening.

Secondary hypertension. Elevated blood pressure caused by, hence secondary to, certain diseases or infections.

Semilunar valves (sem-ee-loo'nar). Cup-shaped valves. The aortic valve at the entrance to the aorta and the pulmonary valve at the entrance to the pulmonary artery are semilunar valves. They have three cup-shaped flaps which prevent backflow of blood.

Septum. A dividing wall. The atrial or inter-atrial septum divides the left and right upper chambers of the heart; the ventricular or inter-ventricular septum divides the left and right lower chambers.

Serum (see'rum). The fluid portion of blood remaining after cellular elements have been removed by coagulation. It differs from plasma, which is the cell-free portion of uncoagulated blood.

Shunt. A passage between two blood vessels or two sides of the heart, as when an opening occurs in the wall which normally separates them. In surgery, the operation to form a passage between blood vessels so as to divert blood from one part of the body to another.

Sign. Any objective evidence of a disease.

Sino-atrial node (sy-noh-ay'tree-al). A small mass of specialized cells in the right upper heart chamber which initiate the electrical impulses that give rise to contractions of the heart. Also called *S-A node* or *pacemaker.*

Sodium (soh'dee-um). A mineral found in nearly all plant and animal tissue. Table salt (sodium chloride) is nearly half sodium. In some types of heart disease, the body may retain excess sodium and water, and sodium intake therefore is often limited.

Sphygmomanometer (sfig'moh-ma-nom'e-ter). An instrument for measuring blood pressure in the arteries.

Stasis (stay'sis). Stoppage or reduction of blood flow.

Stenosis (ste-noh'sis). Narrowing of

an opening. Mitral stenosis, aortic stenosis, etc., mean that the indicated valve has narrowed so it does not function normally.

Stethoscope. An instrument for listening to sounds within the body.

Stokes-Adams syndrome. Attacks of unconsciousness, sometimes with convulsions, that may accompany heart block.

Stroke. Also called cerebrovascular accident. Reduced blood supply to some part of the brain, which may be caused by (1) a blood clot forming in a vessel (cerebral thrombosis); (2) a rupture of a blood-vessel wall (cerebral hemorrhage); (3) a clot or other material from elsewhere in the vascular system which travels to the brain and obstructs a cerebral vessel (cerebral embolism); (4) pressure on a blood vessel, as by a tumor.

Stroke volume. The amount of blood pumped out of the heart with each contraction.

Sympathectomy (sim-pa-thek'to-me). An operation to interrupt some part of the sympathetic nervous system. The sympathetic is part of the autonomic, or involuntary, nervous system and regulates such tissues and organs as glands, heart and smooth muscles not under voluntary control. Sometimes the interruption is achieved with drugs and is called a chemical sympathectomy.

Sympathetic nervous system. A part of the automatic, or involuntary, nervous system that regulates tissues and organs such as glands, heart and smooth muscles not under voluntary control.

Symptom. Any subjective evidence of a patient's condition.

Syncope (sing'koh-pee). A faint.

Syndrome (sin'drohm). A set of symptoms that occur together and are given a collective name.

Systemic circulation (sis-tem'ik). Circulation of blood through all parts of the body except the lungs.

Systole (sis'toh-lee). In each heartbeat, the period of contraction of the heart. Atrial systole is the period of contraction of the upper chambers of the heart; ventricular systole is the period of contraction of the lower chambers.

Tachycardia (tak-ee-kar'dee-a). Abnormally fast heart rate; generally, anything over 100 beats per minute.

Tetralogy of Fallot (te-tral'oh-jee, fal-oh'). A congenital heart malformation involving four defects, hence "tetralogy." Named for the French physician who described the condition. The defects are: (1) an abnormal opening in the wall between the heart's lower chambers; (2) misplacement of the aorta so it overrides the abnormal opening and receives blood from both right and left lower chambers instead of only the left; (3) narrowing of the pulmonary artery; (4) enlargement of the lower right heart chamber.

Thrombectomy (throm-bek'tohmee). An operation to remove a blood clot.

Thrombolytic agent (throm-boh-lit'ik). A substance which dissolves blood clots.

Thrombophlebitis (throm-boh-fleh-by'tis). Inflammation and blood clotting in a vein.

Thrombosis (throm-boh'sis). Formation or presence of a blood clot (thrombus) inside a blood vessel or the heart.

Thrombus. A blood clot which forms inside a blood vessel or the heart.

Thyrotoxic (thy-roh-tok'sik). Pertaining to abnormal activity of the thyroid gland.

Toxemia (toks-ee'mee-a). The condition produced by poisonous substances in the blood.

Toxic. Pertaining to poison.

Tricuspid valve (try-kus'pid). A valve made up of three cusps or triangular segments and located between upper and lower chambers in the right side of the heart.

Uremia (you-ree'mee-a). An excess in the blood of waste materials normally excreted by the kidneys.

Vagus nerves (vay'gus). Nerves of the parasympathetic nervous system which extend from the brain through the neck and chest into the abdomen. They slow the heart rate when stimulated.

Valvular insufficiency. A condition in which valves cannot close properly and permit backflow of blood.

Vasoconstrictor (vas-oh-kon-strik'-tor). Vasoconstrictor nerves, one part of the involuntary nervous system, can, when stimulated, cause blood-vessel walls to contract, thus narrowing the passage and raising blood pressure. Chemical substances, including adrenalin, stimulate the muscles of blood vessels to contract and are called vasoconstrictor agents or *vasopressors*.

Vasodilator (vas-oh-dy-layt'or). Vasodilator nerves, part of the

involuntary nervous system, cause muscles of blood-vessel walls to relax, thus enlarging the passage, reducing resistance to flow and lowering blood pressure. Vasodilator agents such as nitroglycerine, nitrites and other chemical compounds cause relaxation of the muscles of the vessels.

Vaso-inhibitor (vas-oh-in-hib'i-tor). An agent or drug which inhibits action of the vasomotor nerves. When these involuntary nerves are inhibited, the muscles of blood-vessel walls relax and blood pressure is lowered. Nitrite compounds are examples of this type of agent.

Vasopressor (vas'oh-pres-or). An agent or drug which contracts blood-vessel walls, raising blood pressure. Also called *vasoconstrictor*. Adrenalin is an example.

Vein. A blood vessel which carries blood from some part of the body back to the heart.

Vena cava (vee'na kay'vah). The superior vena cava is a large vein carrying blood from the upper part of the body (head, neck and chest) to the right upper chamber of the heart. The inferior vena cava is a large vein carrying blood from the lower part of the body to the right upper chamber. Plural is venae cavae (vee'nee cay'vee).

Venous blood (vee'nus). Unoxygenated blood, carried by the veins from all parts of the body back to the heart.

Ventricle. One of the two lower chambers of the heart. The left ventricle pumps oxygenated blood through the arteries to the body. The right ventricle pumps unoxygenated blood through the pulmonary artery to the lungs.

Ventricular septum (ven-trik′you-lar). The muscular wall di-

viding left and right lower chambers of the heart.

Venule (ven′youl). A very small vein.

Index

263